BREAST CANCER

BREAST CANCER
A Nurse's Journey From Diagnosis Through Reconstruction

ELAINE EMBREY, R.N.

Foreword by Sue Ellen Cooper

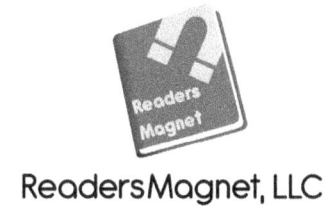

ReadersMagnet, LLC

Breast Cancer
Copyright © 2018 by Elaine Embrey, R.N.

Published in the United States of America
ISBN Paperback: 978-1-948864-38-1
ISBN eBook: 978-1-948864-39-8

All rights reserved. No part of this publication may be reproduced, stored in a retrieval system or transmitted in any way by any means, electronic, mechanical, photocopy, recording or otherwise without the prior permission of the author except as provided by USA copyright law.

The opinions expressed by the author are not necessarily those of ReadersMagnet, LLC.

ReadersMagnet, LLC
10620 Treena Street, Suite 230 | San Diego, California, 92131 USA
1.619. 354. 2643 | www.readersmagnet.com

Book design copyright © 2018 by ReadersMagnet, LLC. All rights reserved.
Cover design by Ericka Walker
Interior design by Shieldon Watson

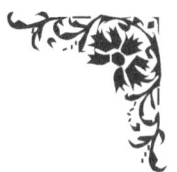

I would like to dedicate this book to my family,
who stood by me throughout my journey and
encouraged me to write "my story."

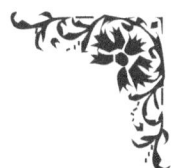

A SPECIAL THANK YOU GOES to Sue Ellen Cooper (*Founder of the Red Hat Society*) who, from miles away in California, held my hand from my diagnosis through reconstruction and shared her faith with me along the way.

Thank you to my twin sister Marge for being just that—my twin sister. You were (and are) always there for me.

I'd like to thank everyone who literally came together in prayer from around the world—Some I know personally, while there are many others whom I will never meet this side of Heaven. You were all part of my circle of prayerful support.

And most of all, thank you to God for giving me the opportunity to grow in my faith while carrying my cross.

Acknowledgements

Ron—my supportive and loving husband, who totally understood my journey

Scott—our eldest son, who was always concerned and as close to us as the phone

Sue—our daughter-in-law, whose love and compassion were so evident

Jeff—our youngest son, who constantly reminded me that I was in his prayers

Hilary—our daughter-in-law, who encouraged me with the success story of her aunt

Sherri—my only daughter, who will always be "my little girl"

Todd—who frequently called and always knew when I needed a "grandchildren fix"

Our grandchildren: Brendan, Kassidy, Morgan, Aaron, Brady, and Brooke, whose love, homemade cards, and hugs kept me going throughout my journey.

I would like to thank my breast surgeon, Dr. Carlotta Maresca; my plastic suregon, Dr. Thomas Beird and his nurse Dee Ann. You always gave me time, compassion, and encouragement.

I would also like to thank my nephew, Brad, who spent hours with me, while editing my book and would not let me give up. My gratitude also goes to Brad's wife, Nancy, and to their children Alison and Joshua, who sacrificed the time that Brad spent with me on those beautiful Sunday afternoons. You all hold a special place in my heart.

Foreword

Having had many nurse friends, it has been my experience that these people are—almost without exception—true caretakers and generous givers. But, even among them, Elaine Embrey stands out. Elaine and I have been corresponding with regularity for several years, and I have been privy to her entire breast cancer ordeal—beginning with the first hint of something suspicious (in June of 2008), through her tests, waiting periods, diagnoses, surgeries, false alarms, accidents, agonized decision-making processes, and, finally, joyful celebration.

Throughout the process, she has demonstrated a determination to face all of it with a positive attitude and upbeat outlook. Even while sharing the gritty details of her diagnosis and treatments with me, she continually expressed deep concern about how the effect her ordeal had on those around her, especially her family. She has steadfastly continued to socialize and enjoy life, keeping herself on an even emotional keel as much as possible, as part of her campaign to encourage others as well as retain her own enthusiasm for life. She had leaned hard on her belief in God and has constantly sought the prayer support of others, including her family, friends and other Red Hatters, including me, who share her Christian faith.

A review of the hundreds of emails that we have exchanged over the past months reveals her concern—arising very early in the process—that she would be able to make a "silk purse out of a sow's ear" by charting the path of her own suffering, thus creating a roadmap for others who must follow her into similar troubled waters. She knew that tapping into her nursing experience and medical knowledge would allow her to offer broader knowledge and a more thorough understanding of the medical processes than that of a "civilian." This book offers plenty of those things.

But she has gone beyond these: she has also shared intimate moments and disclosed her deeper personal struggles. Knowing that there are spiritual and emotional dimensions to cancer, as well as physical ones, she has opened her life to others. This book offers a valuable gift to all who are willing to accept it—a true, personal story loaded with practical nuggets of information, spiritual encouragement and practical wisdom from a nurse who has been there—and survived.

Sue Ellen Cooper
Founder of the Red Hat Society

Preface

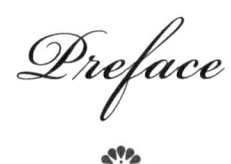

I REMEMBER A TURNING POINT as I was going through my journey. I never asked, "Why did this happen to me?" But I did ask, "Why did this happen? What was I supposed to learn from this? What can I do to create a happy ending to this story?" In other words, "How can I take lemons and turn them into lemonade?"

I kept telling everyone how much I was learning as I was going through this whole experience. I was shocked that there was so much I didn't know about breast cancer and the various treatments for it. I felt compelled to share my newly acquired information with others.

I remember one day, when I was thinking about how much I was learning on my journey. I also realized how much I learned the hard way. If I had been more educated on this subject beforehand, would it have been any easier? I thought it would have, at least in some respects. Dealing with the unknown is the most difficult thing to do. Once you know what you are dealing with, then you feel like you have a "handle on it" and you are more prepared to do whatever you have to do at that point and time.

One day, I simply said, "I'm going to write a book! I'm going to write a book about my experience so that I can help others through their journey." I thought that people would laugh at me, but as I shared my sincere desire to write about my experience in order to educate other women, more and more people encouraged me to do it. They would say, "Who could do it better than one who has been down that road themselves?" Since I am also a nurse, it gave it more credibility.

I remember telling my daughter, Sherri, that I was writing a book. She responded with, "Well, that's right up your alley." Sherri knows that I e-mail everyone and share all kinds of things that happen in my life. She knows that I'm a detail person, who has a difficult time saying anything in ten words or less. So, instead of laughing at me, she encouraged me to write a book—story. Her approval meant a lot to me

My husband was behind me all the way from the first time I mentioned it to him. He thinks that I'm a walking encyclopedia of medical information anyway. So when I told him that I had to write a book, he said, "Go for it!"

My goal was to share what I learned with other women who were on the same journey I was, were about to go through what I was going through, or who knew someone who was traveling the same path. With breast cancer cases on the rise, it's time to make more people aware of it and to encourage more people to support the Breast Cancer Awareness programs. We NEED to find a cause and a cure.

CHAPTER 1

The Diagnosis

❋

I will never forget that day, Thursday, July 31, 2008, when I woke up in the recovery room after my lumpectomy. My husband Ron, my twin sister Marge, and my Aunt Helen were there with me. My breast surgeon, Dr. Carlotta Maresca, a beautiful woman and a breast cancer survivor herself, appeared. I was still somewhat under the effects of the sedation that I had received, but I remember her standing there, appearing to be elevated on a cloud or something but looking at me with total compassion.

My sister asked her how the surgery went. She looked at me and said, "Not good."

The words, "Not good," echoed through my head. I repeated those words, "Not good?"

She said, "They were abnormal cells. We will have to wait until Monday for the pathology report to find out for sure."

I asked, "But you expect it to come back as malignant?"

She said, "Yes," For some reason, it's more difficult to say the word, "cancer," than it is to say, "malignant." So at first, you say, "malignant," and eventually, "cancer" becomes part of your everyday vocabulary.

Being a Registered Nurse myself, Dr. Maresca knew that I wanted her to be totally truthful with me, and she was. I was instructed to call the office on Monday at 3:00 p.m. for the pathology report. My husband and I had plans to go to our friends' house in Oakville, Ontario for the weekend.

We met Barry and Carol 42 years ago on our honeymoon in the Bahamas, and we had gotten together with them at least once a year ever since. Our families grew up together. We went to each other's children's weddings, and when they lost their 35-year old son to a massive heart attack a few years before, we went there to grieve with them. We would not break that tradition just because I had to wait until Monday to get the final diagnosis.

Carol, who is also a Registered Nurse, suggested that we come a day later in case I had any problems after surgery. We agreed and confirmed our plans to go there on Saturday morning and return on Monday. However, we did go to a neighborhood get-together on Friday evening, where everyone brought a dish to pass. We had just moved into our new condo three months earlier, so this was a chance to meet our new neighbors and take my mind off "the big wait."

We met the neighbors in front of the pond and had a very nice time. Some of the neighbors has already heard of my surgery, so they greeted me with big hugs and wished me luck. I told them that I totally expected the pathology report to come back, confirming our suspicion of the breast cancer, so we would just have to wait for the report and then go on to do what we had to do next. More hugs followed throughout the evening, and they all sent us off with their promise of prayers and good thoughts. We went home, went to bed, and left for Canada the next morning. I was feeling good, knowing the prayers, love and support would continue throughout my journey down this new path.

Barry and Carol greeted us with warm hugs and compassion, but we did not spend the weekend laboring over what might lie ahead. We had a wonderful time just being with our friends, who by now have become more like family to us. Their surviving son,

Chris, came over on Monday morning before we left, to see us and wish me well. We were sent off with more warm hugs and good wishes. I was asked to call and let them know what I found out later that day.

Since it took 1/2 hours to get through customs at the border, we were not home yet by 3:00 p.m., when I was instructed to call for the results of the anticipated pathology report. We pulled over to the side of the road and into a small shopping center parking lot, and I called on my cell phone. I thought I was very calm and had everything under control, but I must have been more apprehensive than I even let myself believe because I had to re-dial after hitting the wrong numbers the first time. When I finally got through to my breast surgeon's office, I told the receptionist who I was and why I was calling. I was put on hold, while she got the doctor. I felt tension, as I waited for "my turn" to get my report.

A couple minutes later, Dr. Maresca came to the phone. She said, "Hi Elaine, the report came back as malignant, just as we had expected and talked about after your surgery. It showed a Low-Grade Carcinoma with fibrocystic changes and hyperplasia," This was the first time she used the word, "carcinoma."

Hearing the word "malignant" was shocking enough, but now, hearing the word "carcinoma" was reality. I had cancer! At that time, the word "cancer" became a part of my vocabulary and part of me. It was still a shock, but I was not going to let it get to me. I was going to be strong and handle this with dignity. I was not going to get my family and friends all upset over this, so if I could handle it, they could handle it. Right? I was going to be an example to everyone to show them how something like this could be handled without getting everyone anymore upset than they had to.

Being a Registered Nurse, and having worked in surgery for the last ten years of my career, I saw how apprehension or calmness could be contagious. In scary situations, where things didn't go totally as planned, if the doctor remained calm, then so did everyone else in the operating room. However, if the doctor started yelling and losing control, it affected everyone else in the operating room the same way. This was my chance to show everyone that I was in control and that everything would turn out fine.

However, when you are diagnosed with cancer, many questions go through your mind. *Is this really happening to me, or is it a bad dream?* I went faithfully to my annual pap smears and mammograms, yet it was still happening to me. I was told that the office would set me up for an MRI of both breasts, which is routine before breast surgery for cancer to see if any other lumps or suspicious areas are found. All I wanted at this time was to get into any hospital that I could get into, as soon as possible in Saginaw. I just wanted to get rid of the cancer, once and for all. *Tell me where I can get in first, and I will be there.*

As luck would have it, Dr. Maresca was going on vacation for two weeks, but while she was gone, I would be able to get my MRI completed. Then she would have the results to go over the findings and discuss options. At this point, I just wanted to get this over with…whatever we decided to do.

It's the wait that is the most difficult part of this journey. Once you hear the word, "cancer," you just want to say, "Get it out of me now!" I would have climbed up on my dining room table, if that meant that someone would do my surgery that day. You just feel this urgency to "get it over with."

On August 12[th,] I had my MRI of both breasts, which was a bit of a challenge being inside that tube for so long. But I prayed every minute I was in there. I was cold so I asked for a warm blanket. That proved to make things feel too close, so I asked for the blanket to be removed. That, in itself was freeing. By the grace of God, I made it through the MRI and was now looking forward to my appointment with Dr. Maresca to go over all the tests and make some serious decisions.

On the following Monday, my husband and I met with Dr. Maresca in her office. She confirmed the diagnosis of "invasive ductal carcinoma" (the most common type of breast cancer which involves the milk ducts of the breasts). She also confirmed that I had "carcinoma in situ" (a lump in which the cancer is totally contained). The cancer had not spread, or metastasized, outside of the lump at that time. I was very fortunate.

She also did a biopsy of the dense area, which was evident in my mammogram two years in a row. The biopsy of this "density" in the left breast showed abnormal cellular changes and cysts, but no cancer was identified in that specimen at that time.

My interpretation of those "abnormal changes" was that if those cells were abnormal and changing, then I wanted to get rid of them as soon as possible and before they turned cancerous. In my mind, I was not comfortable leaving any part of the left breast tissue, which may be in danger of causing more problems in the future.

My lump was never seen in the mammograms, extra views, or in the ultrasound that I had when they called me back for an additional views. When I asked Dr. Maresca why the lump did not show up in the mammogram or in the ultrasound, she said, "Mammograms are not perfect. It may have been hiding behind the density."

If the radiologist, who reported that no lump was seen on either the mammogram, the extra views, or in the ultrasound, had not taken the precaution of requesting a biopsy of the "density," I would have gone for another year with breast cancer, undetected, while it continued to spread. Thank God for this cautious female radiologist.

I also experienced something different after all my testing this year. After my routine mammogram, the extra views, and the ultrasound of the breasts, I received a letter from the radiologist. It informed me that my tests showed finding(s) that would require additional imaging for a complete evaluation. The letter also stated that most such findings are benign (not cancer.) However, I was advised in each of these three identical letters to contact my physician to discuss the findings and to schedule an appointment with them for follow-up evaluation. Follow-up was recommended within seven days.

I had to go back for additional views after my routine mammogram the year before, but I never received a letter like that. Perhaps it was a new practice this year? Who knows? In any event, I was not going to tag myself with a diagnosis of cancer with no solid proof. So, life went on and I did my best to remain calm until the next step in the process.

Thinking back in time and recalling everything that led me to where I was now in my health issue, I remembered going for my annual pelvic exam and pap smear on April 30th. My gynecologist asked me if I had felt any lumps in either breast. I told him that I thought I felt a lump in my left breast recently while taking a shower. However, when he checked me while I was lying down flat on the examining table, he couldn't find it, and neither could I.

Since that was the answer I wanted to hear, I didn't insist that I felt a lump and I didn't drive myself nuts by probing and poking to try to find it after I got home. I had several fatty tumors removed from my arms and legs in the past so I was trying to convince myself that it was probably another lipoma. Another thing that kept me relatively calm was that I was scheduled for my annual mammogram on June 2nd (a little over a month later) so that would be more reliable than my suspicions, or so I thought.

I went to have my mammogram, extra views, and ultrasound. All this time I was convincing myself that many women go through this and find out eventually that there is no cancer. I was NOT going to get myself all upset over nothing.

As I was going through the process, step by step, my memory again took me back to one year prior, when I went for my mammogram and then was called back for the cautious extra views.

After those extra views I received a call from my gynecologist's office. The nurse said that my mammogram was perfectly normal. I had a problem with the term "perfectly normal." I tried to be calm but firm as I said, "Listen, I'm a Registered Nurse and I KNOW that everything is not 'perfectly normal'. I saw the films on the view box, and I saw a red circle around the area 'in question' on one film. I also saw a red arrow pointing to the same area on another film. I know that this area 'in question' must have been addressed in the narrative report. I'd like to know what that narrative report said."

The nurse was very kind and went to get that narrative report and came back and read it to me, word for word. It said that it showed fibroglandular tissue, which is basically what the breast is made of. I thanked her and went for another year, thinking that everything was fine and so did my doctors. However, they would pay particular attention to that area the next year when I returned for my annual mammogram.

One year passed and here we were this next year, going through the same steps. But this year was different in that it went a few steps further. After my extra views and ultrasound this year, my gynecologist called me on my cell phone, as I was having lunch in a restaurant with my husband, my sister, my Aunt Helen and her soon-to-be new husband. We were celebrating Helen and Terry's recent engagement when my phone rang. I got up from the table and walked to a quieter place in the restaurant where I could hear better.

My gynecologist was so kind and reassuring as he told me that there was something suspicious on my films this year and that to "play it safe," he suggested a biopsy, so he made the appointment with Dr. Maresca (Breast Surgeon).

On July 2nd I went to Dr. Maresca's office for a pre-op visit to discuss that area in question and the suggested biopsy. I remember telling Dr. Maresca that there was no lump, but I did have an area of density, which had been there the year before but was not there two years ago.

She examined my left breast and then looked me right in the eyes and said, "There IS a lump, and it HAS to come out!"

I agreed with her but again I convinced myself that it was probably a fatty tumor, which most of my immediate family members had the misfortune of forming in their later years. Why would I think anything differently now just because this one was in my breast? My twin sister had two lumpectomies, one in each breast, a few years before. Both of my sister's lumps proved to be fatty tumors, so I just knew that mine would also be a lipoma. Now it was my turn to have a lumpectomy (removal of the lump). They were also going to do a biopsy of the suspicious dense area.

Whenever anyone asked me how I could be so calm during this wait, I would tell them that when I worked in surgery and took care of women coming in for a lumpectomy, I would calm them down by first asking them if they believed in God. Of course, at a time like this, they all believe in God. Right?

Next, I would tell them that if they prayed, and they all said they did, then why not just trust that God was there to get them through this? I assured them that 80% of these lumps are benign, so why not assume that they were in the majority, and it was benign also? If it was not benign, they would have plenty of time to worry about that later on. Why waste the time and effort getting all upset about this now, when they don't even have proof that it's malignant yet? This seemed to help most of my patients somewhat, so I took the same advice.

I also felt responsible for showing my husband and children that I was just fine and that this tumor was most likely benign, like the majority of tumors are. I had them all convinced that I was fine, so when my three children asked if they should come into town for my surgery, I told them that it was not necessary to take a day off from work for this. I assured them that their Dad would call them with the news after my surgery.

My daughter Sherri, who works second shift at a dance studio, nearly one hundred miles away from us, came in at midnight the night before my lumpectomy. We stayed up for a couple of hours, talking and getting caught up on everything. Her visit meant more to me than she ever knew, but I felt bad that she had to drive such a long way so late at night, after teaching ballroom dancing for several hours. She was going through a divorce at the time, which was much harder on me then dealing with my breast issues. I needed to see my "little girl" to know that she was doing all right. She left the next morning after kissing me good-bye.

Our eldest son, Scott, is an engineer who lives in Troy, Michigan and works in the Detroit area. I assured him also that I would be just fine, and it was not necessary to come in for my lumpectomy. I also assured our youngest son, Jeff, who lives in Grand Rapids, Michigan, and works as a Purchasing Agent, that I was just fine and that their Dad would call them with the news after I got out of surgery. Everyone was fine with that.

It was different for my twin sister Marge and my Aunt Helen who decided that they had to, and *wanted* to be there with Ron. Helen and Marge are both nurses, so like all people of our profession, they wanted to hear the results from the surgeon and be there to ask any questions they might have. Of course, they would also support both me and Ron through this entire experience. That's just what nurses do.

The lumpectomy took place on July 31st as planned. There would be many emotional ups and downs as I traveled this journey.

Now, fast forward to August 18th. There I was in Dr. Maresca's office with my husband, going over all the test results and pathology. There was no doubt that we were dealing with breast cancer. There was a cancerous tumor and a density, which was changing cells. This was not good. Something had to be done now; a decision had to be made.

I asked Dr. Maresca what my options were. She said that if I wanted to keep my breast, then I could go through six weeks of radiation, or I could choose a mastectomy. She assured me that either choice had the same prognosis. One wasn't any better than the other; it was up to me to decide.

Fortunately, the night before that, Ron and I discussed my options at home. I was leaning toward a mastectomy. I did not want radiation or chemotherapy, if I didn't have to have either one of them. I also did not want to have one breast removed and wonder when and if I would get cancer in the other one.

I asked Ron how he felt about having a wife with no breasts. He said that he supported any decision that I thought was the right one for me. Knowing that his mother and many others had gone through this twice, I said that I didn't want to go through this again. I wanted a bilateral mastectomy (both breasts removed), and I was okay with going through the rest of my life with no breasts. I was 64 years old, not some young chick, whose breasts are more important to her at this stage in her life.

Ron supported my decision, and I totally expected him to go along with whatever decision I came to after weighing all the options. After all, I was a nurse, so Ron respected my opinions when it came to making medical and/or surgical decisions. He's told many people that I could be a doctor, but I believe that nursing was the right career for me. I was no doctor.

I remember Ron's mother going through breast cancer twice, and both times deciding on no reconstruction. I have to admit that reconstruction after a mastectomy was not that popular at the time of her surgeries. However, I remember like it was yesterday, when she told me what decision she made. She said that her doctor came back with this comment, "Well, Norma, you have your head on straight, so I believe that you are all right with your decision." Remembering how bravely she went through two separate mastectomies, I wanted to feel that I "had my head on straight" also. However, this was all to be discussed with Dr. Maresca the next day. Here we were again…hurry and wait.

CHAPTER 2

Making the Final Decision

❂

Here we were in Dr. Maresca's office, thinking I had it all together and having made my decision. I was proud of myself having it all figured out, or so I thought, and going into that office with full confidence in the choice I had made. I told Dr. Maresca that I wanted a mastectomy but I wanted both breasts removed. I didn't want to have one breast left hanging there. I asked her if I could that.

She said, "Yes."

I asked her if insurance would cover a bilateral mastectomy in my case. She assured me that it would. Then I told her that I was all right with living the rest of my life with no breasts. I told her that I could handle that psychologically. Then there was a big pause, or a loud silence, if there is such a thing.

Dr. Maresca carefully and gently, said, "Oh, Elaine, are you sure?" She went on to say she knew that I cared what I looked like, and she thought that I'd be much happier with reconstruction. It would make me feel "more normal." Then she turned to Ron and asked him how he felt about it.

I have to say that she caught him off-guard, but he quickly responded with, "Well, we actually talked about this last night, and I told Elaine that whatever decision she made was fine with me. It was her decision."

Then I recalled what I heard from someone else, whose friend's husband was asked the same question by his wife. His response was something like, "You can live without your boobs, but I cant live without you." WOW! What a statement! I was assuming that my husband felt the same way, and I believed he did.

Then Dr. Maresca told me that some women think that they don't want the reconstruction, but then they come back in a year or two, and they've changed their minds. After much discussion, I looked at Dr. Maresca, whom I admire so much, and said, "Well, you have been through this yourself. I respect your opinion, and if you went through it and are happy that you did, then I guess I can do it too. I trust you."

Next, Dr. Maresca said that she just had a surgery cancellation for Wednesday, two days later, and if I wanted the time, it was mine. I looked at her and at Ron and said, "I'll take it!" Even though the opening was at another hospital across town, I wanted to go wherever I could get in the soonest.

Dr. Maresca told me that she had to check with Dr. Beird, the Plastic Surgeon. She worked with Dr. Beird on most of these cases, which involve breast reconstruction, and if he was available to see me that day, then we could go ahead with our plans of doing the surgery two days later. Dr. Beird would be the one to insert the expanders after Dr. Maresca did the mastectomy. She went out to make the phone call and came back, telling me that he could do it. Then she took us out to see her scheduler to check to see if that time was still available or if someone else had taken that slot already.

As luck would have it, the slot was still open, so I took it. I hugged the scheduler and said, "Oh, thank you, thank you!" I don't know if anyone before me ever got that excited over getting a surgery time that led them to hug the scheduler, but I was so happy. "Thank God!" I thought. Things were suddenly moving fast, which was good for me—a Type "A" personality who wants everything done yesterday.

We left Dr. Maresca's office, went across the street for a quick lunch, and came back for an appointment with Dr. Beird, the plastic surgeon. He agreed to see me first thing in the afternoon. I couldn't believe how everything was falling into place. I guess "it was meant to be," as the saying goes. We were supposed to meet my twin sister Marge for lunch after my appointment, but now we had more important things to do. Things were beginning to happen, and that was exciting in its own way. I called Marge to bring her up-to-date on things, and off we went to our nexxt appointment.

Dr. Beird's office was just two doors away from Dr. Maresca's office. How convenient! Within five minutes or so from when we entered his waiting room, we were called into the examining room. We sat there for a few minutes, waiting for Dr. Beird to come in. I was on the examining table, and Ron was in a more comfortable chair. As I sat there, sort of nervous, but trying to remain composed, I looked around the room, noticing some pamphlets in holders on the wall. They were for nasal reconstruction, breast reduction and a few other topics, but there were none in sight that said, "Bilateral Mastectomy with Reconstruction."

I sat there, with my feet crossed and swinging below me somewhat, as I do when I feel apprehensive. I remembered doing this same thing with my feet, before my lumpectomy. I was in the radiology room before surgery, waiting for the radiologist to do a "needle localization," which is a procedure done in which a wire is placed under the guidance of x-ray through the skin and right to the tumor. This was done so that when you go into the operating room, there would be no question as to where the tumor was located.

As I sat there that day, waiting for the radiologist to come to the room for the procedure, the radiology technician noticed my anxious feet. She gently put her hand on my feet to stop me from swinging or shaking them. Until then, I didn't think I was nervous. Remember, I was a nurse; I was strong; and I "had it all together," or so I thought.

When I went to my plastic surgeon's office, the nurse came into the room, asked some questions and then took pictures of me standing in front of a sheet with nothing on from the waist up. First, she took a frontal view and then a side view. All I could think was, "This must be somewhat like it feels when you go to the police station for 'mug shots.'" However, instead of holding a number, I think I held a paper with my name on it. This helped to keep that identified picture in my chart, to see what my breasts looked like before the mastectomy. I felt uncomfortable during this 'photo shoot,' and almost asked, "Should I smile?" But I didn't say anything. I did what I was told to.

Shortly after that, Dr. Beird entered the room and introduced himself. He confirmed that he had talked to Dr. Maresca, and knew that I was coming in that day to see him. He opened up a box, which contained expanders and silicone breast implants, and asked me to hold an expander and feel the silicone implant. Being a past surgical nurse, I had seen and felt these before but, I would be the recipient of these foreign objects this time, *not* my patient. I never thought I would ever be in this position—getting breast cancer and needing a mastectomy.

There was practically no history of breast cancer in my family. My dad's mother died of breast cancer at age 60, and my mother's sister got breast cancer when she was in her 80's. I never dreamed I would be the next to get breast cancer.

Dr. Beird explained that he would be inserting the expanders after Dr. Maresca was finished with the mastectomy. Expanders are put under the chest muscle. They have a tube with a port, through which the saline is injected for each expansion. The plastic surgeon locates the insertion site by moving a magnet over the skin to find the partially metal port below the surface. After locating the port, the spot is marked with ink, and a needle, which is connected to a big syringe filled with saline, is inserted into the port. As the saline is injected, it stretches the skin and muscle to prepare for the permanent implant.

Once the tissues have been stretched to the desired size for the implant chosen, it must stay stretched for 3 1/2 to 4 months. This procedure is necessary, because the skin has memory and wants to go back to where it was before. This made sense to me, after having three babies and knowing how stretched out my skin was during the pregnancy, yet it eventually all went back to how it was pre-pregnancy. Now, I understood why there would be a time period between the final expansion and the final surgery.

The final surgery is 'the exchange,' This is when they remove the expanders and replace them with the final implants, either saline or silicone. Oh, if I could only push some 'fast forward' button to speed things up. I was ready to say, "Let's get started!"

I knew from my friend, Heather, who had just recently gone through this phase, that it was a long process. But, as the saying goes, "Sunday's coming!" I just had to take it one step at a time. There would be a light at the end of the tunnel; however, I was about to learn what it really meant to be a patient. Patience is indeed a virtue which *this* Type "A" personality would have to learn to practice.

After all the explanations about how the surgery would be performed, Dr. Beird asked me the big question, "What cup size do you want to be?"

This immediately reminded me of my sister Jackie, who lives in Naples, Florida. She is one year older than my twin sister and I, and she is always giving us (the nurses) medical advice or opinions. She had been calling me on a daily basis by this time, and one thing that kept echoing in my head was, "Just think, Elaine, you can now be any size you want to be. Go for it!"

I looked at Dr. Beird, purposely not looking at my husband, because I wasn't sure if I wanted to know how he would answer that question, and I said, "Well, I'm wearing a 'C' cup now, but it's a 'C—Long,'"

He smiled, as I'm sure that he'd heard that before. I mainly wanted to end up with a couple of "perky girls," as my sister-in-law

Jan called them. I told Dr. Beird that I wanted to be a "C" or whatever he thought was appropriate for my size frame.

He said, "Well, you have to go to at least a 'C' to have definition." I never thought of it that way. I thought that if I were looking for definition, I needed to go to the dictionary. The word "definition", took a whole new meaning. I told him to use his judgment and do what he thought was right for me.

After I left his office, I wondered if I should have set limits. Oh well, he had been doing this for a long time, so he should know what was right for me. At least that is what I was counting on. We left his office and would now have to wait for the surgery to be done two days later. Wow! Things were moving right along. I was all set to have a double mastectomy in two days.

I was told that I would be getting phone calls from the hospital to pre-admit me and to get my medical and surgical history. They told me the usual things: nothing by mouth from midnight on; take only prescription drugs; no Aspirin or any drugs that would increase my bleeding time; no contact lenses in; no make-up, etc. My surgery was scheduled for 12:30 p.m., and I was to report to the hospital two hours earlier. The reality of it all was coming out loud and clear.

On the way home from the plastic surgeon's office, I called my twin sister Marge and all three of my kids. I convinced my kids that I was doing just fine with all of this, and there was no reason for them to be there at the hospital on the day of my surgery. Our daughter Sherri was leaving that weekend for Minneapolis, Minnesota for a dance competition with one of her dance students and was swamped with extra practices in order to tie up loose ends before the competition.

Our son Jeff was leaving for a much-needed family vacation which had been in the works for quite some time, and our son Scott, (the engineer) had some big jobs going on at work that he was overseeing. He was going to try to drive up to Saginaw after he got out of work, the day of my surgery. I told all of them that I would be coming home on Thursday, the day after surgery, so I would not be there very long. Jeff, who was on vacation, was going to try to come up the following weekend after I was home for a while. That would be just fine.

My sister Marge, who had just had rotator cuff surgery two weeks before, and my husband Ron would be there with me and would call my kids after surgery to let them know how everything went. Because my brother Ken was working second shift and six to seven days a week, it was just about impossible for him to get the day off. My other two brothers, Larry and Don, and sister, Jackie, all live out-of-state. I talked to all of them on the phone and assured them that I would be just fine. After all, what could they do for me while I was in surgery for several hours? They all assured me of their prayers, good thoughts and/or support. I needed that more than anything else.

CHAPTER 3

Hurry and Wait

❈

Here I was. It was Monday afternoon. I had just seen my breast surgeon and my plastic surgeon, and I was on the surgical schedule for Wednesday, which was two days later. Again I wanted to hit the "fast forward" button somewhere to get me to the day of my surgery. What could I do to help the time pass by more quickly?

I kept myself busy, e-mailing friends and family and/or talking to them on the phone I had been sending out e-mail "Updates on Elaine" each time there was something new to report. My kids were worried, but by my staying relatively calm, they would also be able to stay relatively calm.

I continued to tell everyone that I would be just fine. I was going to get rid of the cancer once and for all, and by having a double mastectomy, I would never have to go through this again. My mother-in-law had gone through two mastectomies, seven years apart, and she did just fine. I could do the same. I just wanted to have my surgery and get on with life.

There were no real tears up to this point. I didn't even cry when I was initially told that my tumor did not look good and that it was probably malignant. I was so proud of myself for being so much in control. My sister helped me get dressed to go home after my lumpectomy, shortly after we were told that we were most likely dealing with cancer. As soon as they drew the curtains around us to give me privacy, Marge hugged me as she was crying. I choked back a couple of tears but then pulled myself together and off we went.

The nurse walked me out to the car, and I thanked her and said, "Good-bye." I told one of the nurses that I would be back, but I don't think she caught that. I used to work at St. Mary's and this was their off-site surgical center where I volunteered after I retired from the main hospital. I knew many of the nurses who worked there and talked to them before I went into the operating room. However, the nurse who discharged me was not one of them, so my friends didn't know the outcome of my lumpectomy. I was escorted out to Ron's car, and we drove home in a different frame of mind than we were when I arrived a few hours earlier.

Marge and I were together a lot during this waiting time. She had just had rotator cuff surgery two weeks before my scheduled mastectomy, so we joked together and kept the conversations light. We even joked about the tattoos that I would have when the time came to make new nipples. There we were, both RN's, and neither of us knew that part of the reconstruction was to make a new nipple, also known as a tattoo. I was learning something new every day. Jokingly, I told Marge that maybe instead of nipples, I might choose to have Mickey on one breast and Minnie on the other. We laughed. I didn't know how intricate breast reconstruction was going to be. This was a whole new subject to get to know.

My grandmother had one breast removed for cancer when I was about eleven years old, so she went the rest of her life with only one breast. I remember when she came to live with us for the last few years of her life, seeing her stuff a handkerchief in her bra cup on the side that had no breast. This was her way of feeling more "normal."

Then there was my mother-in-law who more recently had her surgeries. Each time she chose to have just the mastectomy and used an external prosthesis, which she inserted into a pocket of her bra to make her feel and look more "normal." She shared with me one time that when she told her doctor she was all right with not having anything else done, he replied, "You have your head on straight, so I believe that you are okay with your decision." We all admired how bravely she went on with the surgery and the rest of her life, having two separate surgeries seven years apart.

I wanted to be brave too, and I thought that I "had my head on straight," so initially, I was willing to have both breasts removed and just use the external prostheses. I never gave it a thought that I would ever go through breast reconstruction. My knowledge of that procedure was very limited, even though I was a Registered Nurse who worked surgery the last ten years of my career. I had seen mastectomy surgeries, but I never witnessed the placement of the permanent implants, nor did I know much about the stretching of the skin and muscle to prepare for the implants.

All I knew was that I didn't want to wait to have another diagnosis of breast cancer sometime down the road. I kept telling myself that all I wanted was a bilateral mastectomy so that I wouldn't ever have to worry about going through this again. I would be just fine. I was hoping and praying that the cancer had not spread to my lymph nodes, so that I would not need chemotherapy. I also chose a mastectomy over radiation, I didn't want want to damage good tissue, in case I ever needed to have open-heart surgery for my leaking tricuspid valve. This was my decision, and I was not about to change my mind.

When I saw my plastic surgeon on that day, two days before my surgery, he told me I was going to have pain, and it would not be from the mastectomy. A mastectomy is basically a painless surgery, but the pain I was going to have would be from what he had to do to prepare for the implants. His work involved working with the muscle, and whenever you work with muscle, you are going to have pain.

I told him that I understood, but I had never experienced that "cut-muscle" type of pain before, so I really didn't know exactly what he was talking about. He told me that I would have medication to help me with the pain. We discussed what pain medication he would order, since there are so many that I cannot take due to the way I reacted to them in the past. We decided on Tylox, which was one that I had not tried before. One more decision was made, and now I was ready and just had to wait for Wednesday to come.

I came home and sent another update via e-mail to all of my friends and relatives, who were waiting for more information. To me, keeping busy with these updates was calming, and it also gave me something to do with the time. Each time I sent out an update, I'd get lots of e-mail responses in return, so it kept me busy but in this case, it was a blessing because it helped fill idle time.

In addition to my family and close friends, whom I was trying to convince that I would be just fine, I developed a deep relationship with someone very special in my life. I had been e-mailing her almost daily since my diagnosis in July, when the lump was discovered. This special lady is Sue Ellen Cooper, the founder or "Exalted Queen Mother" of the Red Hat Society.

For those of you who have never heard of the Red Hat Society, it is an organization (or disorganization, as we call it, since the rules are "loose" in some respects), in which you earn the right to join when you turn 50 years of age. This, in itself, gives you the right to wear the red and purple outfit and join the Red Hat Society along with thousands of other ladies who have reached that age also.

At this time, there are more than one million Red Hatters all over the world. We have decided to *celebrate* growing older, rather than dread it and have stood by our motto of : "All of my life, I've done for you…Now it's time do for me." In other words, this was the time in our lives that we vowed to find time to have fun. We were committed to making time to go out and do fun things with other ladies who felt the same way. While some women in the past used to get depressed when they reached their fiftieth birthday, many women now look forward to it because they will then be qualified to join this special group.

Marge and I started our own chapter of the Red Hat Society in 2002 and chose our name of "Prominently Purple Red Hatters." The founder of each chapter is known as "Queen," but since my sister and I are Twin Queens, we call ourselves "The Tweens." Since we have been involved in Red Hat activities over the past several years, we have had the pleasure and opportunity to meet "The Exalted Queen Mother," Sue Ellen Cooper from Fullerton, California, in person a couple of times. Eventually, we planned to go to the International Red Hat Convention in Nashville, Tennessee in 2007. It was just before leaving for that event that I had my annual mammogram and found out for the first time that I had this density in my left breast.

I chose to keep my plans of going to the convention and have my additional films to investigate this density after we returned from the convention. I had told Sue Ellen about my situation, via e-mail, before I went there, and she said that she would pray for me. We talked about it briefly in person while we were at the convention, and I assured her that I would be having the extra films shortly after I returned home. I remember telling her that whatever was there would still be there when I got back home, so I was not going to cancel my trip to the Opryland Hotel that I had paid for in advance. I looked forward to being with my red-hatted sisters. I was going…end of discussion.

I did have those extra views after I returned home from the convention. However, the additional views did not show a lump, so I was asked to return in one year for my next annual mammogram. When they convinced me that I had no lump, I was glad that I had not canceled my trip. Marge and I had a wonderful time at the convention, and then we met up with my sister Jackie fron Naples, Florida and my sister-in-law Susie from Fairfield Glade, Tennessee. After that, we went to see my niece Shelly, who lives in Conyers, Georgia. We had a wonderful and fun time with the girls. When we returned home, I had to face reality again. However, I was so glad that I got to experience a huge International Convention at the Opryland Hotel, where over 3,000 Red Hatters were in attendance. It was an awesome experience.

When I went for my next annual mammogram, suddenly they were concerned about this density again, which had not been there two years before. I e-mailed Sue Ellen and asked for her prayers once more. Somehow, we connected, and over the next several months there were numerous e-mails going back and forth. We shared our family backgrounds, our dreams, our feelings on motherhood and our joys of being a grandma. We found out that we had a lot in common even though we were totally different individuals.

I found out that Sue Ellen grew up in Massachusetts, which totally shocked me; I thought that she had always lived in California. She remembered walking to school in the cold winter, breaking through the ice, arriving at school with soaked shoes and socks and lying down and making angels in the snow. It was fun to reminisce about our childhood and the things that we had in common. Oh, how I wished that we were neighbors and could sit down now and then and just chat, but I will probably never leave Michigan, and Sue Ellen will never leave California.

Over the next few months, Sue Ellen also shared something special with me—her faith. She got me to dig down into my soul and feel the presence of God, when I was trying so hard to carry too much of this burden by myself. I wanted to be strong, but I found out that turning my burdens over to God was not a sign of weakness. It was simply admitting my human limitations. While I was thinking I was so brave, she read between the lines and encouraged me to admit my limitation and let others help me get through this. I remember part of one of her letters, which read:

> *"As I have already said, I admire your courage and your determination to spare your loved ones as much as anxiety as possible. But, dear Elaine, my prayers are more for you than for them. Courage can only take you so far. You need the love and care of Jesus, and I am praying that you can sense His presence right now. I can tell you that whenever I have desperately needed Him, He has made me very aware of His support. You know He's with you."*

Sue Ellen was absolutely right. I could not get through this alone. I needed to let Jesus be my co-pilot. Together we could handle it. I told her about Pat and Bob, friends of ours, who came over and gave me a beautiful silver cross that had a silver tab on it with the Biblical inscription, "I can do all things through Christ who strengthens me" (Philippians 4:13). I was wearing that cross and tab continually. I would have to take it off to go to surgery, but it would go back on to be a constant reminder to me that I was not alone. I could either keep it, or if the occasion came when someone else needed it more than I did, I would feel free to pass it on to that person. I did not know at that time where the cross would end up, but it did go to someone else a few months later. That person kept it for a couple months and then gave it to someone who needed it more than she did. What an amazing experience that was.

Sue Ellen remained faithful to me in prayerful support and in sharing her faith with me, which made it easier for me to share my faith with her. She helped me realize that it's time for me to be "the patient" and not "the nurse". I had to let go of that control. It's not easy for nurses to switch roles like that. We like to be in control. Sue Ellen helped me switch roles by saying the following: "I hope that you are able to realize fully how many lives you have obviously touched. All that you have given out is coming back to you. When people care about you they are anxious to be there when you need them. Don't be shy about letting them care for you. It is good for them to be able to show their love. Your turn to care for others will surely come again." I needed to hear that in order to "let go."

Sue Ellen also mentioned that she was glad that I was having reconstruction. She said that the women she knew, who have had it, are glad they did become because it's less of a radical change. That made me feel better and not feel vain because I was going with the reconstruction. Sue Ellen also told me about a friend of hers who used to do a lot of runway modeling and teach classes on make-up and clothing. She said something that made (and still makes) a lot of sense. "I take care to look the best I possibly can every day, and once I've done that, I can forget about myself and focus on others for the rest of the day."

I had a big decision to make regarding reconstruction, but now I was comfortable with my final decision. I guess I needed that affirmation more than I realized. I told Sue Ellen that my beautician fit me into her busy schedule the day before my surgery to give me a body perm, in case I was unable to use my curling iron for a while after surgery.

I also had my nails done that day. I told her it was not a totally vain thing but rather a "for me" type of thing. It makes me feel better on the inside when I feel "together" on the outside. I'm hoping that others, who have to make this decision of reconstruction versus no reconstruction, will have a friend like Sue Ellen to help them feel better about whatever decision they make. It's a personal decision for each and every one of us, and one decision isn't any better than the other.

I received another opinion while seeking help in making my decision. I e-mailed our good friends, Margaret and Leeds, asking them if they thought it was a vain thing to have reconstruction after a mastectomy. Leeds wrote back saying,

> *"No matter what you choose to do, some 'dit' will think you should have done something else. Do what I do: please yourself. Make a list of pros, another of cons. Throw away the list and do what feels best to you. That's always the right choice. Hey, this is all about you and Ron—but he'll want you to do what you are happiest with."*

That's what I needed to hear. Case closed.

The night before surgery, many e-mails and phone calls came in, wishing me luck and assuring me of their prayers and good wishes. I went to bed feeling loved and watched over. I knew that the next day would be a big day, so I hoped to get a decent night of sleep.

CHAPTER 4

My Support Group

I CANNOT BEGIN TO TELL you all the support that was coming in. The phone calls, the numerous e-mails, the hugs, the promises of prayers, etc. I was not alone, and that felt so good. We had just moved into our new condo three months earlier, yet our builder and his whole crew were praying for me and wishing us well. His office manager gave me many hugs to help me through the whole ordeal. Our realtor and her associate were holding us up in prayer. My entire family and a multitude of friends were assuring me of their concern, love, and prayers. It was awesome.

A nurse classmate of mine was calling me daily at this time. I remember her first call. She was crying and saying, "Sista, I don't want to lose you." We call each other, "Sista" and I jokingly call her my "Southern Sister." We were in the nursery together after we were born and our mothers were roommates. Little did we know that eighteen years later, the three of us, Dee and the twins, would end up in the same nursing school together and become like sisters. She now lives in Louisiana but comes to Michigan yearly, and the three of us always get together while she is in town. We call her husband "brother-in-law." They are like family.

I also received a lot of support and love from my new neighbors, Doug and Jean. Jean is a Registered Nurse, who made numerous phone calls to me and was so caring to both me and my husband Ron. She was also my medical consultant, when I needed her expertise. Doug is a Lutheran minister, who had been keeping up with my situation through my e-mails and wanted me to know that Ron and I were in his prayers. One day, as I was reading my e-mails, I was pleasantly surprised to see one from Doug. The email shared a prayer from Doug's collection of pastoral resources. This prayer was exactly what I needed to hear at this time. It talked about how much we want to be in control of our own destiny, but at the same time, God offers to lead us and bring us through any situation we are facing if we would just trust Him. After letting these words sink into my heart, I realized that God was speaking directly to me.

Being married to a nurse, Doug knew very well that nurses like to be in control. Yet, here was another reminder that it was time to "let go and let God."

Our pastor, Fr. Bert Gohm, and Assistant Pastor, Fr. Kevin Kerbawy, were keeping tabs on me also. We had recently had them over for dinner, and they were very caring and concerned about me. Our pastor said that when I knew when my surgery was going to be, he would like to give me the sacrament of the sick and anoint me. I told him that I would like that. He preferred to do it in church on a Sunday to have some of the church community in attendance to help pray for me. Unfortunately, I went to see my breast surgeon on a Monday, and there happened to be a cancellation on Wednesday, two days later, there would be no more Sundays on which to go to church to have the Anointing of the Sick with members of the congregation present. That made me feel really sad because I really wanted this to happen, however, I knew that God was looking out for me because I was on my prayer chains all over the United Stated. How could I not feel good about my outcome?

The day before my surgery we were invited to our good friends, Don and Win's for dinner. I jokingly called it "The Last Supper." We had been through a lot together with this couple over the years.

This time it was my turn to be facing surgery, so we were invited over and accepted the invitation. I was asked to say the blessing before the meal. I somehow got through it, but it was a bit emotional. Our friends had both faced some serious surgeries before, so they knew that there was always the element of the unknown, which caused a bit of apprehension before the actual surgery. However, I was going to beat this thing called, "cancer," so I wanted to have the surgery and get it behind me. I waited patiently long enough. Sometimes I think that the wait is harder on us than the actual surgery. Once you know what the problem is and what you have to do in order to make things better, you just want to get on with it.

My kids called to wish me well. I was pre-registered at the hospital and had my insurance card and driver's license ready to go with me plus my list of daily medications. I had given my health history to the nurse over the phone and was told that they would get the insurance pre-authorization when I sign in at the hospital. I was as ready as I could possibly be. Let the show begin.

I was instructed to take a shower with an anti-bacterial soap the night before as well as the morning of the surgery. I did not need an infection, so I scrubbed with my soap and rinsed off well on the night before and the morning of the surgery. I had never been so clean.

I even paid my bills, so that I would not have to worry about any unpaid bills for a while. I knew it would take a few days to clear my head from all the medication, so I wanted to be call caught up or early in all of my bill payments. It's amazing all the things that go through your head at a time like this. The laundry was caught up, the ironing was done, there was plenty of food in the house and the house was clean. You would have thought that I was getting ready to have a baby, trying to leave everything in order before going to the hospital. There was not much more I could have done in preparation for the big day. I even called my former neighbor, Lee, whom I affectionately adopted as my mother, to talk to her one more time before surgery and assure her that I would be just fine.

That night I knelt to say my bedtime prayers. I didn't know how much sleep I would get thinking about my surgery the next day. I asked God to take care of me, and even though I knew I had breast cancer, I prayed that the lymph nodes would be clean so that I would not have to have radiation or chemotherapy. Was I asking for too much? I hoped not. However, I also prayed that I would be able to accept whatever diagnosis I would receive and have the strength and faith to deal with it and accept what I couldn't change. It was at that time that I realized how hard it was to say, "Thy will be done," and really mean it. Most of the time when we pray at a time of crisis, we are really saying, "I want MY will to be done." however, I fully realized that my destiny was in God's hands now. I had to let go. I looked at my silver cross and the Bible verse on it, and I knew I could get through it.

Some people feel a need or compulsion to get on the computer and read everything they can find on breast cancer before making any decisions regarding mastectomy versus radiation. My sister-in-law, Susie from Tennessee, is also a Registered Nurse and works for a radiation oncologist. She encouraged me to do all this research but I just couldn't. There is way too much information, and while I know most of it is good information, I also know that not all of it is up-to-date.

If I were in Susie's position and could run some of this information past my boss before surgery, I may have tried to absorb as much information as I could. However, time was running out, things were moving fast, and I just couldn't spend all the time necessary reading through reams of information, not knowing what was up-to-date and what wasn't. Besides, while watching TV just before my surgery, there was a doctor on one of the talk shows who said this very same thing. Even though there is a lot of good information on the Internet, not all of it is accurate or up-to-date. Time was a factor, so I had to trust that my doctors were guiding me down the right path.

A subsequent e-mail I received from my sister-in-law stated the following:

"When I told you that you may want to look at different types of breast cancer and their treatments on the Internet, it was to help you formulate questions for your physicians. I also said to keep an open mind and try not to let the information from what my doctor calls 'WalMart Parking Lot' influence you. Each person's situation is different. All the information on the Internet can be overwhelming. People deal with things differently. I remember that my mom told me to tell her only what she needed to know at the moment, and for me to get all the information that I wanted, and she'd asked me when she was ready to know more. Many Cancer Centers are starting to offer a 'nurse navigator' to help cancer patients, especially breast, through the system because it can be so confusing. We've just started a program."

Among my support group of friends and family, three separate people sent me or brought me a handmade shawl. One of these shawls came with a pamphlet about 'Shawl Ministry." The pamphlet includes an explanation about why and how these shawls are made and given away to those in need of comfort and solace. It is very moving to read about the many blessings that are knitted into every shawl. The person who is knitting it begins each shawl by saying a prayer for its recipient and continues to pray for that person throughout the making of the shawl. This person also says prayers upon completion of it before sending it along its way. Two of my shawls had purple and/or red in them, which are the colors of the Red Hat Society. Being presented with these shawls was a very touching time for me. These shawls, like my silver cross with the Biblical inscription, can be eventually passed on to others who need them. I am so blessed to have so many loving family members and friends to help me along my journey.

By the time the day of the surgery came, I was ready and wanted to move forward. Many women were going to my same breast surgeon and plastic surgeon, and they all seemed very satisfied with them. I felt comfortable with them also and was anxious to just get my surgery behind me and then concentrate on the recovery. I didn't want any uncertainties to consume me or add to the apprehension and stress that I had already experienced. Although I appreciated everyone's concern and suggestions, I realized that in the end, it had to be MY decision and one I was comfortable with. I had to trust my doctors, which I did.

Ironically, as it seemed, one of the Prayer Chains that I am on, frequently comes with a Bible verse at the end of the prayer requests. One of the e-mails I received recently, quoted Proverbs 3:5-6, "Trust in the Lord with all your heart and lean not on your own understanding; in all your ways acknowledge Him, and He will make your paths straight." That was about as appropriate and timely as it could be.

CHAPTER 5

The Day of Surgery

I woke up early that morning and went into the bathroom. It was while I was in the shower that I realized that this would be my *last* shower with breasts. I wondered what it would be like to come home without that part of my anatomy. As I lathered up, I washed for the last time, and a flood of tears suddenly came pouring out. I hadn't really let my emotions get the best of me before this, but now, I literally sobbed as I finished my shower. I rinsed off, got out of the shower and began to dry off. Again, it hit me that this was the last time I would be drying off this part of my body. I wanted that day to get here as soon as possible, but now that it was here, I experienced a reality check.

Ron came into the bathroom as I was getting dressed, took one look at me and knew that this was a difficult time for me, seeing my red eyes from crying so hard. Without saying a word, he took me into his arms and held me close, as we both burst into tears. I felt his body shaking, as I'm sure he felt mine. We just stood there, sobbing and holding each other. We both needed that. We had been strong for each other long enough. Now, it was time to give in to our human weaknesses and let it all out. It was so cleansing. I thank God for that moment and for a man who loves me enough to cry with me at a time like this.

At 6:29 a.m. I sat down at my computer and wrote the following letter:

> *Good morning everyone,*
>
> *Well, we're in the countdown stage. We'll be leaving for the hospital in less than three hours. I ask for your continued prayers. I will be coming back home tomorrow. I will be back at my computer as soon as I can. In the meantime, please keep the prayers coming. I still need them. I'm trying to say, "Thy will be done," but I find myself still praying for a cure. I am also hoping that my lymph nodes are clean so that I won't have to go through chemotherapy.*
>
> *Ron and Marge will be with me at the hospital. Scott is coming after he gets out of work. I have to be at the hospital at 10:30 a.m. for a 12:30 p.m. surgery time. Thank you to all who have been praying for me, sending cords, e-mails, flowers and your loving support. Soon we will know what we have to deal with. I still have my silver cross from my friends Pat and Bob, which has a tab inscribed, "I can do all things through Christ, who strengthens me." (Philippians 4:13). I wish I could keep it on throughout surgery, but I cannot wear any jewelry. I am hanging in there. Please stay with me in prayer.*
>
> *Love,*
Elaine

Minutes later I received this e-mail from my cousin Judy, who is also a Registered Nurse and works at the hospital next door to where I was to have my surgery:

> *Morning Elaine,*
>
> *You don't need the cross, since you have Christ always with you! Just remember His words and He will provide the strength you need. He has chosen you to have this journey for reasons only known to Him. He will be your guide and you will learn whatever lessons you will need to learn. You are a pillar of strength and*

inspiration to me. I have to work this morning, but He has let me sit here and read your e-mail this a.m. Obviously, I am running a little behind but this is what He wants me to do. I am sending my prayers and love to you! I will hold you in my heart.

Hugs great lady!
J.

Judy will never know how much that letter and her gift of taking time to write it meant to me. We draw strength from each other. Her letter helped me to get into the right frame of mind to be able to move on, feeling confident that whatever I found out after surgery, I would be able to deal with it. It's the unknown that adds to the apprehension.

At 9:00 a.m., our Pastor, Fr. Bert, called. He was wondering if we were still home. I told him that we would be leaving in one hour. He asked me if I would like to be anointed. I told him that I would love that, so he said he would be right over. He was not kidding. In what seemed like minutes, he was at our door. I let him in, and we all went into the living room. Ron sat on the couch next to me and was asked to put his hand on me. He put his arm around me as Fr. Bert said some prayers and then anointed me with the holy oil. I was so happy that I could receive this sacrament of the sick before going into surgery. As soon as Fr. Bert finished, I saw Ron take his glasses off to wipe away his tears. I put my hand on his and assured him that I would be okay. He responded with, "I need help." At this time, I hurt more for Ron than I did for myself.

As we walked Fr. Bert to the door, we both thanked him for taking the time to come over to do this for us. He seemed happy to be able to give this blessing. After he left, I went over to my neighbor, Jean's house. I told her that I needed one more hug, which she gave me and assured me of her prayerful support. Doug had already left for work, but I knew he would be praying for me also. I had so many prayer partners that I knew that I could get through whatever I had to. I was so fortunate.

I checked the computer one more time and found an e-mail from our Realtor Sheli. It read,

> *Good Morning Elaine!*
>
> *You may already have left for your surgery, but I just wanted to let you know that I have been and will continue to cover you and your family with prayers. You amaze me with your strength and positive attitude, and I have such a great amount of respect and admiration for you. God Bless You Elaine and Ron and Marge. Good luck today and know you have a huge following of prayers covering you.*
>
> *See you soon!*
>
> *Love,*
Sheli

Is it any wonder why I felt prepared physically and spiritually for my surgery? I was on more prayer chains around the world than I ever knew. I also received an e-mail from my twin sister Marge which said:

> *Everyone who prays is already praying and will continue. All you have to do is close your eyes and allow God to guide the hands of your surgeons.*
>
> *Love and continued prayers,*
Marge

I responded with, "I understand. 'Let go and let God.'"

After I left for the hospital, the following e-mail came in from Fr. Kevin:

> *Hi Elaine,*
>
> *By the time you read this, I hope you have GOOD NEWS and that the surgery went WELL and you are already in the process of continuing healing. You will be in my special intention at Mass this evening at St. Hedwig's. I've been praying for you*

this morning. I picture God holding you tenderly, smiling at you dearly and saying, "All will be well."

Love,
Fr. Kevin

Another e-mail arrived after I left for the hospital and it would be waiting for me to read after I returned home. It was from Sue Ellen Cooper.

By the time I send this, you will be in the hospital—hopefully with the surgery over with. I know it will be a while before you're back on the computer, but please know that you are in my prayers often, all day. I know that we must pray for God's will to be done, but it doesn't come easy for anyone.

Love,
Sue Ellen

When it was almost time to leave to go to the hospital, I felt a dandy headache coming on. I took an Imitrex pill, which I usually take for Migraine headaches. It didn't help, so I took another one about fifteen minutes later. I still had no relief, so we left for the hospital and went up to the pre-op area, where I went through the normal admission procedures. After the nurse was finished asking all of her questions and filling out all of her papers, she went to get Ron and Marge and let them come into my room to stay with me until it was time to go to the operating room.

Just before 12:30 p.m., the surgical nurse came to get me. She let Ron and Marge follow next to me until we got to the elevator. They both gave me a good-bye kiss. Marge was crying by this time, which caused me to shed a few tears. I pulled it together, and off we went on our separate ways. I was going to the pre-op room, and Ron and Marge were going to the surgical waiting area. Little did we know at the time that they would not be allowed to see me until nearly seven hours later.

Shortly after arriving in the pre-op room, I met a female anesthesiologist, and I was asked all those questions regarding my health history, medications, reactions to medications, etc. I don't remember what her name was, but I do remember that she never smiled. She was serious and very business-like. It was that experience that reminded me of something I had heard long ago, which was something like, "You may not remember a person's name, but you will never forget the way they made you feel." How true!

After answering all the necessary questions, the nurse came to start the IV on me. Since the cancer was in my left breast, she tried to start the IV in my right arm but was not successful. I was so dehydrated from not being able to eat or drink anything since the night before. Dr. Maresca, my breast surgeon, came into the room and stood next to my cart. She smiled warmly at me and asked how I was. I told her that I had a terrible headache. The nurse told her that she could not find a vein on my right side and asked her if it was all right to look on my left arm. Dr. Maresca gave her permission to start the IV in the left arm.

As the nurse was working hard to find a suitable vein, Dr. Maresca stood by my side and held my right hand. Just feeling the warmth of her hand, holding mine was calming. She didn't have to say a word to convey her compassion. Isn't it strange how by merely standing there, quietly holding a hand can speak volumes? A breast cancer survivor herself, she knew exactly how it felt to be lying in the pre-op room, knowing that when you came out of surgery, both of your breasts would be gone. I could feel her compassion and her gentleness. I needed that more than anything else at the time. She stayed by my side until the IV was started, and they were ready to take me into the operating room.

Because they usually give you some Versed intravenously, just before you leave the pre-op room to help you relax, I never remembered entering the operating room. Those drugs usually hit me right away, and I'm "down for the count," as they say. Well, this time was no exception. I have absolutely no recollection of entering the operating room or of being transferred to the operating table. The next thing I knew, it was seven hours later, and I was in my hospital room in the post-op section. I would stay in the hospital overnight and then go home the next day, which is all they allowed.

I had no idea of what my family was going through during those seven hours that we were separated. Dr. Maresca came out at 2:30 to tell them that the mastectomy part of the surgery was finished and went well. She said that she removed three lymph nodes from the left side and one from the right, and they all looked good. She would be very surprised if they came back showing any cancer. She also said that Dr. Beird was doing his part of the surgery, preparing me for the reconstruction.

At 4:00 p.m. Dr. Beird came out to talk to my husband and sister to report that all went well, but that I had very thin chest muscles. Therefore, they would have to be more cautious with my expansions. Consequently, there would be less saline injected at each expansion because of my thin muscles. If he went too fast, the muscle would tear and "roll up like a shade." Well, we certainly didn't want that to happen.

He told my family that I would be in the recovery room for about an hour, and then they would be able to see me. However, I would be in some pain and probably nauseous for some time. He also told them that if I was not ready to come home the next day, all the nurse would have to do is call him, and he would change the diagnosis to allow me to stay a second night. It was much easier to control pain and nausea in the hospital then at home. Ron was relieved to hear that they had the option of letting me stay a second night, if necessary.

Now, they were in another waiting mode waiting to see me. Five o'clock came and went. Six o'clock passed by. Finally, at 6:15, Ron went to the desk to ask what was going on. The woman looked in the computer and told him that I was still in surgery. Well, he knew that wasn't right, so at 6:30 he asked if someone could call the recovery room to ask what was going on. He wanted me to know that I was not alone, and that they were there. They did just that and were told that I was all right, but they were waiting for a room.

All this time, Ron and Marge were told nothing, which caused a lot of apprehension. A few minutes later, Ron asked if he could go to the recovery room to see me. They told him that I would be going to my room soon. Finally at 7:05 p.m. they were told that I was in my room.

By this time, our son Scott had just arrived at the hospital. Ron waited for him to go up to see me while Marge went right up. Shortly after that, Ron, Scott and my brother Ken arrived in my room. I don't remember too much except for a lot of confusion and moving me around to make room for another patient to come into my room. I remember thanking everyone for coming and giving good-bye kisses before they left. It had been a long day for Ron and Marge, and the extra tension didn't help. They went home, and Ron took my place at the computer and sent out an update after making a few phone calls to our family members who were not there. What a day that was!

When Scott came, he brought homemade cards from his two children, Brendan and Kassidy. I was in no shape to read them until I got home. However, when Marge was sitting at my bedside at the hospital the next day, she picked up the cards and read them.

Brendan (age 10 1/2) wrote,

> *Get Well Soon. I love you so much, and losing you is such an unbearable feeling.*
>
> *Love,*
Brendan

WOW! That was quite a statement.
Kassidy (age 9) wrote,

> *Dear Grandma,*
>
> *I love you so much and I know that you'll get better! Even if you don't, you'll still be with me in the heart. GET BETTER SOON.*
>
> *Love,*
Kassidy

Both of their cards were filled with little hearts. They were so special. I had no idea all the thoughts and emotions that our grandchildren were experiencing during this time. Their parents told them ahead of time that I was going to have surgery for breast cancer, but that I would be okay. Well, these kids knew everybody that has cancer doesn't necessarily get better, so they were worried.

Our two grandchildren from Grand Rapids sent their cards through the mail.

Aaron (age 7) wrote,

> *Dear Grandma,*
>
> *I hope you get better.*
>
> *Love,*
Aaron

Morgan (age 10) wrote,

> *Dear grandma,*
>
> *Get Well Soon!!! I hope you feel better soon. I really miss you. I hope I can see you soon.*
>
> *Love,*
Morgan

Our youngest two grandchildren, Brady (age 5) and Brooke (age 4) were too young to make cards, but they had their own little questions, and they were happy to come see me after I got home from the hospital and had some recovery time. Seeing and hearing from those six grandchildren was the best medicine I could have received. Also, the love, prayers and support from my family and friends helped me through some pretty tough days. I am very fortunate to have all those people in my life.

All these key people in my life reminded me of a story about a train ride, in which people get on and get off the train, along your journey. Some stay longer than others and become very significant to you, while others come and go and are forgotten. However, each one serves a different purpose. Isn't that true?

I have very good friends, whom I have not known that long, like Doug and Jean. I also have long-term friends like Barry and Carol, whom we met on our honeymoon and have become like family over the years. I have a friend by the name of Marilyn, whom I have known since first grade. She has stood by me through all of my tough times and prays for me every night. Whenever I was scared, she sensed it and gave me encouragement and assured me of her prayers. We have seen each other through some pretty trying times over the years. Our bond has continued to grow over many years.

Then there are my walking friends at our condo complex, whom we call the "Walkie Talkies," and the three couples that we travel with and have over for dinner once in a while. We also have a whole group of Marriage Encounter friends, who are very special and faithful prayers warriors, too. All these people are so very important to me and have helped me whenever I needed them. Let's not forget my Red Hat Sisters who are there whenever there is a need, and the "Soup Man" and his wife who faithfully show up at your doorstep with a fresh pot of soup without ever being asked. I could go on and on and on. So many people have gotten on my train and each and every one of them has served a purpose in my life.

Some of my contacts are strictly through e-mailing, but they are there for me and as close to me as my computer. This is what modern technology has done for us. I also have family members, whom I see a lot and some whom I rarely see, but they were all with me on my journey. I am indebted to each and every one of them. It's overwhelming when you try to think of all the people that have gotten on and off your train throughout the years.

I felt that Sue Ellen Cooper held my hand throughout my journey, and she said that she could almost feel my pain. In one of her e-mails, she wrote,

> *"The prayers continue, almost non-stop. I feel almost as if I am going through this with you—which is silly, as I can't possibly understand the physical issues or the anxiety. But, nonetheless, I do feel that way. The Bible tells us to bear one another's burdens, and this must be a glimpse of how that feels."*

My friend, Heather, had been through the same things that I was going through. She was my best source of information because she went to the same breast surgeon and plastic surgeon. She always said it like it was and always assured me that I could handle whatever I was faced with.

I was also in close contact with the daughter of one of my nurse classmates, Kathy. Kathy and Dave's daughter Cheri was diagnosed with breast cancer that was more advanced than mine, but her attitude was a great inspiration to me. Someday, I want to meet Cheri in person and rejoice together as breast cancer survivors.

And then there is my twin sister Marge. Talk about bearing one another's burden…well, let me tell you. She has been with me through thick and thin. She spent the entire day at the hospital with Ron during my surgery, which was two weeks after her surgery to repair her full-thickness tear to her rotator cuff. I was with her during her surgery and recovery period, and then she was with me. We're both nurses, so we were able to help one another with our showers, dressing changes, getting dressed, etc. Being a twin is an experience that I wish everyone could have. There is nothing that compares to this unique bond. I remember growing up together when we were young. If one was scolded and cried, the other twin cried also. If one fell and cried, our parents had two crying twins to deal with. Talk about bearing one another's burdens you have no idea.

CHAPTER 6

Coming Home

THE DAY AFTER SURGERY was one I prefer not to remember. Now I know why these e-mails keep coming, trying to get people to write their congressmen to pass a bill to allow women to stay in the hospital for more than one night after a mastectomy. Since I chose to have to reconstruction, it meant that I would have pain for a while. It was a totally different story than if I had just had a mastectomy without the reconstruction. In my mind, and in the opinion of my husband and sister, I was not ready to come home in 24 hours. I was in pain, I was nauseous, and I felt very light-headed. However, my allotted time was running out, so I was being prepared to be discharged that evening. When we asked if I could stay for one more night, we were basically told that if I stayed…I paid. No thanks! We were out of there.

It was 9:30 at night when I was discharged, so we could not get my prescriptions filled until the next day—neither the pain medication nor the antibiotic. The nurse was not allowed to send even one of each pill home with me. Luckily, my sister just had rotator cuff surgery and had the same pain pills and antibiotic that I was prescribed. She gave me some to get through the night until our pharmacy opened the next day. In all fairness to my discharge nurse, he did apologize for having to send me home, feeling as bad as I did. He honestly felt that he was doing what he had to do. His hands were tied, or so he thought. However, my nurse neighbor, Jean talked to her Nurse Manager about my situation later, and the conclusion was that I should have asked to talk to the supervisor. I've learned that you really need to be your own advocate in situations like these. I should have known that I could do that, but I was too sick to think. Live and learn.

When a mastectomy patient goes home, she has two Jackson Pratt drains, one coming from each breast site. You are told to empty these drains daily by opening the bulb to release the suction, empty them into a cup they supply you with, then measure the drainage and record it on two separate sheets of paper. When the drainage is finally down to 30 cc per 24 hours, the drains can come out. The tubing, which is attached to those bulbs, is sewn to the incision line and the tube goes several inches inside the operative site to allow the drainage to come out.

My husband and sister were taught how to "milk" the tubing in case a blood clot formed going from the incision to the bulb. I was also sent home with a bag full of dressings, some which had a slit in them to go around the tubes and some that went over the tubes connected to the bulb.

My sister was there when the nurse did my one and only dressing change before sending me home. At first they asked Marge to leave the room during the dressing change until she said, "I am her twin sister. I am a Registered Nurse, and I will be doing her dressing changes at home, so I need to see what it involves." Because she spoke up, she was allowed to stay, but I wondered what the average non-medical woman did when she had to go home the day after a mastectomy. Who would change her dressings? There was no mention of a Home Health Nurse follow-up to see how everything was going at home. No wonder my friend, who had her surgery one month before mine, felt like she was thrown out to the wolves. I felt sorry for her when I listened to her stories. I understand it's dictated by the insurance companies, but it's too bad that more exceptions are not made. Since I was not allowed to be one of those exceptions, I have some good advice for anyone who asks what they should take with them when they go to the hospital. I tell them to "take a nurse"—and I mean it!

It was good, in a way, to get home again, but adjustments had to be made. I tried sleeping in my bed the first couple nights, but that just made it difficult and painful to get up out of bed. Then my friend Heather reminded me that sleeping in a Lazy Boy chair was more comfortable and did not cause all that pulling on the stitches that lying in bed did. So, for the next four weeks, I slept in my Lazy Boy.

From the day I got home from the hospital and continuing on for several days, my friends and family were at my rescue. Food, like you would not believe, was filling my refrigerators. Flowers, plants, gifts and love filled my house. My house looked like a florist's. My dining room table was end-to-end with floral arrangements and the rest of the house was filled with plants—huge plants.

One of my friends sent me a beautiful, ceramic angel and another friend and her husband, whom we knew since high school, brought me a ceramic angel with a pink ribbon for breast cancer awareness. Other gifts I received from friends were a pink ribbon lapel pin and a beautiful bracelet made with metal pink ribbons and pink rhinestones. I even received a black golf towel with a pink ribbon decorating it and a cute little black felt drawstring bag with the pink ribbon. I believe that most or all of these items, with the pink ribbon decorating them, are helping cancer patients or cancer research.

Looking around my condo and seeing all that love and support brought tears to my eyes. Cards kept pouring in daily and filled the top drawer of one of my living room end tables. It was unreal. I even received a piece of Sue Ellen Cooper's own artwork. It was a beautiful painting of a floral arrangement in a vase. I have since had it framed and it is on the wall over the bed in our guest bedroom. I now refer to that room as "The Sue Ellen Cooper Room." She thought that was hilarious and asked if that was like the "Abe Lincoln Room in the White House." I said, "Yes, same concept."

Two days after my return home, our son Jeff, came in from Grand Rapids. It was so good to see him. I was able to visit for a while, but whenever I had to take another pain pill, my head felt weird, I became nauseous, and had to resort to my chair to get some sleep. My cousins, Bill and Monica, came that day also and brought all kinds of prepared food fit for a king. I was really being pampered. I even received a gift certificate for a pedicure from our friends, Bonnie and Joel. Being a surgical patient proved to have some perks, in spite of everything else I had to endure.

As time went on, the doorbell continued to ring and friends and relatives continued to bring food and send flowers and gifts. The mail carrier was also kept busy, bringing dozens of "get well" and "thinking of you" cards. E-mail letters were popping up on my screen like popcorn each time I turned on my computer. So many people were with me in thought and prayer. It was so overwhelming.

As the days went on, we developed our own system of dressing changes, emptying drainage tubes, showering, and dressing. My sister helped me for the first few days, but by the fourth day, I was able to talk Ron through the dressing changes and emptying the drainage tubes. He even remembered how to "milk the tubing" when they got plugged with little blood clots. He listened well, when Dr. Beird explained how to do this after surgery. I was so proud of him.

On the Sunday after my surgery, my fourth day post-op, I decided to go off the strong pain pills and resort to Extra Strength Tylenol and Motrin. I could not stand the weird feeling in my head and the nausea that the strong pain pills caused. First, I alternated the two pills every four to six hours, and then I decided to take one of each every four to six hours. That worked out quite well for me at the time. I was able to not only go to church that day, but I also went to a bridal shower with my sister. This shocked all of my family members, who knew that I had just gone through a double mastectomy and insertion of expanders four days before that.

When the time was right, our Son Scott, his wife Sue and their children, Brendan and Kassidy, came to see me at home. It was so good to see them again. I will never forget Brendan coming up to me ans asking, "Grandma, is it all right if I hug you?" Looking into his crystal blue eyes and at the compassionate look on his face almost brought tears to my eyes. I realized that children need the reassurance that hugging a patient with cancer is not going to hurt them.

I looked at Brendan and said, "Of course you can hug me." As I held him, I could feel the love going from his body into mine. It was a tender, firm, but gentle hug. Brendan is a very sensitive, caring and loving boy and knows how to express it well.

I also gave Kassidy a hug and felt her kindness, love and compassion. Those darling children needed to see that their Grandma was all right and to be reassured that Grandma was going to get better. Unfortunately, it was only a couple of years earlier that they lost a great-aunt to cancer, so I'm sure that *my* diagnosis with breast cancer triggered those painful memories.

Through my experience with breast cancer and surgery, I became very aware of the need for the children and/or grandchildren to know about cancer and surgery. You don't have to go into details about it, but they need to know what is happening. Their age will dictate how much information is necessary. It is good to hug them and let them hug you. Some children may be afraid to touch you at first. They may think that they will hurt you if they hug you. They deserve to hear you tell them how much their hugs and cards mean to you. They need to know that they make a difference in your recovery also.

A couple weeks after my surgery, our son-in-law Todd brought Brady and little Brooke here to see me. They had a new jeep and they were anxious for us to see it. Since they are only 5 1/2 and 4 years old, respectively, they didn't understand exactly what I had gone trough. Consequently, when we went out to the driveway to see their new vehicle, Brady was standing on one of the wheel covers and when I got near him, he jumped off and was flying airborne toward me. I naturally ran to catch him, but OUCH! Todd told Brady that he couldn't do that but I was glad that those little ones looked at me as being the "same old Grandma" as before surgery.

This entire journey had been such a learning experience—understanding what effects it had on me personally and those with whom I interacted. I also learned a lot about the prevalence of breast cancer today. After doing much reading, researching, and hearing stories of other women, I realized that there are way too many cases of breast cancer all around us. What I'm finding out now is that only about 15% of women with breast cancer have a strong family history of breast cancer. The other 85% of them just happen for reasons unknown to us. Things like pesticides, air pollution, and water pollution factor into the picture as well. This is why we need more and more money for cancer research. People are continuing to die from exposure to elements causing various types of cancer and it's time to find out how and why. There is way too much information that we don't know yet. It's scary.

After my breast cancer had been diagnosed and my breasts removed, I needed to concentrate on what my role was going to be in this war against breast cancer. I had months of recovery time, during which I would try to figure this out. There are no clear-cut answers, but there must be some way, I thought, to take lemons and turn them into lemonade. Journaling my experience became not only a way to process everything that was happening to me, but it also became a way that I could help others who might travel down this road in the future.

When I went to see my breast surgeon for my post-op visit after my mastectomy, I got the official report: ALL OF MY LYMPH NODES WERE NEGATIVE! We got rid of all the cancer. Thank you, God!

I cried harder getting the good news than I did when I got the bad news, but that's all right. I would not need chemotherapy or radiation. Instead, I would only need Tomoxifen for five years, and that was up to me to take or not take, since it was believed that I was cured. The Tomoxifen is a drug that keeps the estrogen from bonding with the cancer cells, in case there were any stray cells left. It was left up to me to think about it and decide.

My type of cancer was estrogen receptive, which basically means that estrogen feeds the cancer cells and helps them to grow. I had done that long enough, being on hormone replacement therapy for nearly ten years. It used to be thought that HRT was like a "fountain of youth." It supposedly helped your heart stay healthy, kept your bones from losing calcium, and basically kept your body from aging so fast. Well, now there are newer studies that show that none of this is true. They always knew that there was a higher risk of breast cancer if you were on HRT, but now they are finding out that it contributes more to it than they originally thought.

I begged to stay on my hormones because each of the four times that I tried getting off the hormones, my hot flashes came back every fifteen minutes and night sweats about every hour. I decided that I couldn't live like that and was willing to take the risk of staying on a low dose pill. I'll never know if I could have prevented this breast cancer if I had never gone on hormone replacement therapy, but I don't recommend it to women now, after my diagnosis of breast cancer. It may be safe to stay on it for short-term, but not ten years like I did.

The studies should start showing drastic drops in breast cancer since thousands of women who used to be put on hormones for a long period of time are now only kept on them for a short time or not at all. It would be interesting to see the cancer rates dropping as fast as we watched them skyrocket. Live and learn.

After I had been home for nearly three weeks, I realized that I was feeling worse the third week than I had the second week. *Why was this happening? Was this normal?* I decided to contact the nurse advocate from the health center. Ann had come to see me and brought some literature about mastectomies the day after my surgery. She even gave me a heart-shaped pillow to use in the car between my chest and the seat belt. Fortunately, she left a card with her picture and work phone number on it with the days and hours she was available to take calls. I was still so drugged up the day after surgery that I didn't remember much about what we discussed at the hospital, but I did remember asking for more literature from the American Cancer Society.

Since I was beginning to feel worse than in previous weeks, I looked up this card and called the number. I asked the nurse advocate if I could talk to someone who had gone through the same surgery that I had gone through to find out what was normal and what wasn't at this stage of recovery. Ann told me that she would contact the American Cancer Society to put in my request and that I should be hearing from someone soon.

Well, it took several days, but I did get that call from a woman in Midland, Michigan. We talked for almost half an hour comparing notes, symptoms, and expectations. She was so kind, and I felt so much better after having talked to her because now I knew that having these ups and downs was not abnormal. She assured me it would get better and I would be so happy that I opted for the reconstruction. She, herself, had cancer in one breast and did not have the reconstruction at that time, but a year and a half later, she developed cancer in the other breast. It was then that she opted for the reconstruction and was so happy for the results. This talk greatly encouraged me and I would strongly recommend anyone to seek out this type of help after a mastectomy. There is nothing like talking to someone who has been through what you are going through to bring understanding and peace.

On October 16th we saw an oncologist. She asked me how I felt about chemotherapy. I thought that since I had a double mastectomy and my lymph nodes showed no sign of cancer that I was "home free." She agreed that my prognosis was good. However, it's not the *size* of the tumor but the *type* of cancer that dictates the likelihood of the cancer returning. I could suddenly feel my heart pounding. Was I hearing correctly?

She also suggested using an anti-cancer drug for five years. I was already on Tamoxifen but she switched me to Arimidex since she felt it was a better drug for post-menopausal women. It was a terribly expensive drug because it was relatively new. I did not want to risk getting a recurrence, so I agreed to make the switch. She was going to talk to Dr. Maresca about the switch.

She also suggested sending my tumor to a lab that could test it to see what my chances were of my type of cancer coming back. It was a VERY expensive test (about $3,000.00) and the lab that did this test (Oncotype DX) would check with my insurance company first and then call me to see if I still wanted to go ahead with it. Not every insurance company covers the cost of the test.

My head was spinning as I left the office. I did NOT expect this scare again. However, I agreed to go ahead with the test, even if it wasn't going to be covered by my insurance. What else was I supposed to do? Ron and I left the office speechless. We had received a lot of information that we were trying to process. Another bomb had hit us. We were not prepared for this.

My oncologist also ordered a bone density test and lab work, which was done that day after we left her office. The reason that the bone density was ordered was because anti-cancer drugs are apt to cause osteoporosis (a considerable amount of calcium loss from the bones), so we needed a baseline test to see how dense my bones were to start with. I was already taking a medication called Fosamax for osteopenia (the loss of some of the calcium in the bones). I was hoping and praying that it didn't get much worse, leading to osteoporosis.

The next day on our way to my daughter-in-law Sue's surprise birthday party, I received a call on my cell phone. It was a gentleman from the lab that was to do the Oncotype DX text on my tumor. I just froze as I listened to him.

He said, "Elaine, I checked with your insurance company about covering your test."

My voice was shaking, as I said, "Yes?"

Then he said, "Now listen to what I'm going to say…I am NOT going to spoil your weekend. I checked with your insurance company and I want you to know that your insurance company has agreed to pay 100% of the test."

At that point, I began to cry. I thanked him profusely and went on to the party to have a wonderful time. We survived another stressful event. Money should not have been a factor in choosing the type of care I would get, but when we were talking about extremely expensive drugs and a very expensive test, I didn't know how much worse the situation was going to get.

On November 6th we went back to see my oncologist. She had the results of my testing. The nurse took me into the examining room and took my blood pressure. It was 140/70.

I said, "My blood pressure has NEVER been that high."

The nurse said, "You are probably nervous."

I said, "Yes. I'm VERY nervous."

When the doctor came into the room she sat down at her desk. I was on a chair opposite her and Ron was sitting right next to me,

I felt every muscle in my body tense up as I watched the doctor flipping through pages in my chart. Then she looked up at me and said, "We have your test results. I want you to know that anything under 18% is considered 'low risk.' Your result is 7% so you do NOT need chemotherapy."

At that instant, I began to cry. I said, "Thank God!" Seven proved to be quite a number. It took God seven days to completely create the earth. Now, I can see why seven is a number of completion.

My oncologist got up from her desk, came over to me, and gave me a hug. The suspense was gone. I did not need chemotherapy. What a blessing!

CHAPTER 7

The Reconstruction Process

Healing from having both breasts removed was just the beginning of my recovery. Since I chose the breast reconstruction to be done in conjunction with this, I had a long road ahead of me before I would get to the end of my journey. I had no idea of all that would happen along the way. When I went to my plastic surgeon's office for my first post-op visit, I was told that the scheduler would call me to set up a date for my first expansion. If you remember, the expanders were put in the day that my breasts were removed, and some saline was added to the expanders to get the tissues expanded enough to insert and hold the permanent implants.

Well, as luck would have it, the scheduler didn't call as soon as I expected. When she did, she had the first date available for my first expansion, which was during the time we would be on our vacation out West. We were going to see the different parts of Arizona, including: The Grand Canyon, Zion Canyon, Sedona, Bryce Canyon, Lake Powell, Bell Rock, Montezuma Castle, Cathedral Rock and even Monument Valley in Utah, where they filmed some of the John Wayne cowboy movies. I told the scheduler that maybe this was a blessing in disguise, and perhaps it would be best if I waited until after my two-week vacation to start with the expansions. She agreed, and we set up a date for when we returned home. I still think that waiting until after our trip was the best idea for everyone.

When I went to see my breast surgeon for my first post-op visit, I told her about our planned trip out West. I asked her if I could still go. It would be four weeks after my mastectomy.

She responded with, "Why not? I went to Italy two weeks after my surgery."

Well, that was all I needed to hear. Our trip was a "go." I also asked her about an elastic sleeve that some women wear when they fly in airplanes; due to the altitude sometimes causing lymphedema (swelling in the arms or under the arms). She assured me that since she had only removed three lymph nodes from one side and one from the other, I didn't have to worry about lymphedema.

I had one scare shortly before we left for our trip. I noticed a red area under my left breast and thought it may be the start of an infection. I called my plastic surgeon's office and asked to talk to the nurse, Dee Ann. She told me to come in so that she could check it out.

When she saw it, she said that she was not worried about it, and she was sure it was not an infection. I also told her that when I was stretching, I felt something pop inside. She said I may have popped a suture inside, which was nothing to worry about at that time. I was so relieved and tearfully told Dee Ann about our upcoming trip out West. She gave me a big hug and told me to enjoy myself. I was given a prescription for Keflex to take with me…just in case,

When I went to my gynecologist for a follow-up visit, he said that I could have popped some scar tissue that was forming, but I didn't have to worry about it. I also remember asking my plastic surgeon if I could go on our trip out West. He said, "As long as you don't ride the bulls." That made me smile. Riding bulls was not on my agenda. That's for sure. At any rate, it was nothing to worry about. The trip was on and I was happy. We were all set to go and have a good time with our friends, Tony and Mary Jane.

We climbed mountain trails, did a lot of walking and even rode in a pick-up truck, pulling a trailer load of people over the land where they filmed John Wayne movies. It was so bumpy and hilly, but I had the heart-shaped pillow I had received the day after my surgery. I used it to put between me and my seat belt and off we went. My surgery and my recovery would NOT hold me down.

I have to admit that by the end of each day, my breasts were both throbbing. There was only one time, however, when Mary Jane asked me how I was doing, that I broke down and shed a few tears. She must have seen the look in my face that told her I was hurting. I responded with, "I'm so tired of hurting and taking pain pills every four hours.'

She gave me a big hug, and that's all it took to, "put on my big girl pants and deal with it," as they say.

We had a wonderful time on our trip, and we were so glad that we didn't cancel out just because I had surgery four weeks earlier. I was going to hurt at times whether I was out West or at home, so why not keep busy and take my mind off my health issues during this time? I would use extra pillows at night under my torso as well as under my head and we managed quite well. I was so glad that Dr. Maresca encouraged me to go instead of suggesting that we cancel our trip. We had a wonderful time and made lots of memories with our friends. Some people thought I was overdoing it so soon after surgery, but others understood, mainly Dr. Maresca. The truth is that so much of the recovery and healing time is affected by our emotions. I knew that if I took time to enjoy life with friends and family, I would be on an emotional high, which would certainly help my healing process.

Shortly after we got back from vacation, I went for my first expansion. I really didn't know what to expect. Dr. Beird performed the next procedure exactly how he explained it to me earlier. He moved a magnet over my skin where he thought the post must be, and once found it, he marked it with a pen. Next, he injected several cc's of saline into this marked area. It was a weird experience because I could feel not only the pressure of the saline going into the expander, but I could also feel my chest rise. It hurt as the needle went through the skin and then through the muscle, but that was the worst part.

After he finished doing the two injections, I said, "That wasn't so bad!" I left the Procedure Room and went out to the waiting area where my husband was sitting. I came out smiling and repeated, "That wasn't so bad."

The second expansion, which was done two weeks later, was not bad either. However, I woke up during the night feeling like I had a strap around my chest that was being pulled tighter and tighter. After that experience, I told Dr. Beird about it and he said he would give me some Valium for the muscle spasms. That's what was happening! It was a bit scary not knowing why my chest felt like I had a tight strap around it, but now it made perfect sense to me. My muscles were rebelling from being stretched and were probably wondering what in the world I was doing to them. If I, as a nurse, was wondering if this could be one of the symptoms of a woman's heart attack, I wonder how scared the non-medical person is when this happens to them? I was not having any shortness of breath along with it, so I eventually ruled out a heart attack, but I honestly was surprised at these symptoms when they first began.

The third expansion was a little more challenging. Each expansion was a little different. I squinted my eyes, as Dr. Beird pushed the needle through the skin and then through the muscle. As he was injecting the saline into the expander via the port, he looked at me and said "You know, you're a tough cookie!"

I asked him if some women are able to smile as they are having their expansions. He said, "I see everything from one extreme to the other, believe me!" I'm sure he does.

When I went for my fourth and last expansion, Dr. Beird warned me that this one would hurt, and he wasn't kidding. It didn't hurt right away, but by the time I got home, it was hurting. I had taken some Motrin before I went to the hospital, but that did no good. I went to visit my sister Marge, who lives next door to us, but I had to come home because I was too uncomfortable. I was pacing at her house, holding my breasts, Marge said, "Elaine, that doesn't look good."

I folded my hands and kept them under each breast and asked, "Does this look better, like I'm praying?"

She chuckled and said, "Yes, that looks better." I had to laugh too, even though it was hurting.

I came home, took two Extra Strength Tylenol and took a warm shower, but nothing took away all the pain. After two or three days, I was finally feeling better. I took one Valium each night when I went to bed, and that usually helped me get a decent night of sleep. I discovered that by nighttime, my breasts would be feeling tight due to spasms, but the Valium really seemed to help. Eventually, I was even able to sleep on my side again, which I had not been able to do for quite some time.

Life was getting easier, but I still felt deformed because my expanders were so large and bulging under my armpits and my breasts were way too high. Dr. Beird told me that the permanent implants would be smaller, lower, and softer. I was happy to hear that because, as I told him, I didn't want to look like Dolly Parton. At this time I felt like I was growing "little beach balls" in there. He understood. The expanders were so inflated that if I fell on my face, I was sure that I would literally bounce back up again.

After four expansions, I was the size that we decided was right for me. In fact, at my last expansion, Dr. Beird felt that the right breast was a little larger than the left, so he went back to the right breast and removed some saline, instead of injecting more into the left one. Thank God for small favors.

Since my mastectomy, I was no longer able to wear any type of bra no matter how big it was, because it would cut into my armpits. Here I was, at age 64, going to shop for "cute little under shirts," which were soft, stretchy, and comfortable. Who would have thought I would ever go back to that type of undergarment?

I wasted so much money on all different kinds and sizes of bras, including the sports bra. However, the sports bra was too tight and made my breasts hurt all the time. It was just a matter of trial and error and a whole lot of learning as I went along.

After my fourth and final expansion, I made a HUGE mistake, for which I paid dearly. Since the muscle spasms were really bad for a few days and pain pills didn't help, I decided to use a heating pad over the incision at night to calm down the spasms. I used it on "medium" for two hours and on "low" for one hour plus I had my cotton pajamas on and the flannel cover for the heating pad. In spite of the precautions that I was taking, I managed to get a third-degree burn. I did not feel it happening because the sensory nerve endings for hot and cold were no longer there. Therefore, when I got up in the middle of the night to go to the bathroom, I looked at my incision and found a big blister about the size of a quarter, right on the incision line of my left breast. I panicked and thought it was an abscess, knowing that an abscess meant an infection. I did NOT need this!

When morning came, I told Ron that I was going to have to go to the doctor's office or to the hospital because I thought I had an abscess. I choked back the tears as I saw the look on Ron's face. I was trying so hard to do everything right, but I goofed—big time, I wanted to say, "I'm so sorry," but I was on the brink of crying, so I swallowed hard and called the doctor's office. When the message finally got to Dee Ann, she had the receptionist call me to ask how soon I could get there. I was on my way again!

Dee Ann took me into the examining room and when she saw my blister, she also thought it was an abscess and was ready to send me to the hospital probably for IV antibiotics. She was going out to get Dr. Beird to look at it first. On her way out of the room, I mentioned that I had used a heating pad. She stopped dead in her tracks and said, "That's a third-degree burn!"

The only thing I could think of to say was, "Well, that's better than an abscess, isn't it?" She agreed.

When Dr. Beird came into the examining room, he confirmed the diagnosis of third-degree burn. He told me to keep it covered but to use a blow dryer (on low) to help dry it out, so it would start forming a scab. He also put me on antibiotics.

I went home and soon a scab formed. This scab continued to get thicker and thicker. After four weeks, it had not started to separate from skin. Dr. Beird told me to come back in another four weeks, at which time it was still very thick, not shedding and was now concave (an inward depression). He was afraid that the burn may have gone down to involve the muscle, which, as it was trying to heal, was pulling the scab inward.

Dr. Beird took a deep breath and looked at me. I just knew what he was going to say. My tears were very near the surface, but I didn't cry. He decided that we had waited long enough, and it was now time to be more aggressive. I agreed.

The right thing to do now was to remove the scab in surgery under sterile conditions, and clean out the wound. Then he would do a secondary closure of the incision in order for it to have enough time to heal before my scheduled surgery for "the exchange." This would be when he would remove the saline tissue expanders and put in the permanent silicone implants. The surgery was scheduled for the following Monday and the burn scab was removed. The wound was cleaned out and the scar was revised, along with the scar on the right breast, so they would match. This was indeed the right thing to do. I wanted to keep MY surgery date. Once I was told the date of my final surgery, it became "my date". I did NOT want to give it up. It was another "goal" I wanted to achieve.

When I woke up in the recovery room, the nurse asked me how I was feeling and if I was having any pain. I told her that I was having pain, but it was in my right breast though surgery was on my left breast. Dr. Beird also did a revision of the scar on the right, so it would match the scar on the left. Upon hearing this, I almost chuckled and wanted to ask, "How many people does he think are going to see the scars on this nearly sixty-five year old lady?" But I didn't. I was just glad that my surgeon was a perfectionist, even in "little old ladies".

I saw Dr. Beird three weeks before my anticipated Exchange Surgery, when they would remove the expanders and replace them with the silicone implants. I had to have an extra surgery two weeks before that for removal of the burn scar caused by the heating pad. While I was there for the scab removal, he did some revisional surgery on my scars. I was in good shape now. Everything was healing well; my scars were where they should be; and everything looked perfect. Now all I had to do was meet the nurse, two days before my March 5th surgery, sign some forms for the implants, and I would be all set to go. I was excited that my "exchange surgery" was getting so close.

Dee Ann sent home some papers for me to read and bring with me on my next appointment two days prior to surgery. This was exciting. Dee Ann was such a knowledgeable and caring nurse, whom I looked forward to seeing each time I went to my plastic surgeon's office. I felt free to call her with any questions, anytime. I called her my "life-line," and that she was

I spent over two hours in Dr. Beird's office at the last appointment—one hour in the waiting room and another hour in the examination room. Dee Ann took me into the room and removed a few loose steri-strips from my previous revision of the incisional scars. I was told later that I should remove the remaining steri-strips when I took my shower the next day. Any kind of paper or adhesive tape stuck to me like super glue, so it's no wonder that Dee Ann didn't force the remaining steri-strips to come off. She left those for me to remove after they got wet and softer in the shower. Even though I removed them in the shower the next day, some skin came off with them.

I sat patiently, waiting for Dr. Beird, knowing that when he came into my examining room, I would have his full attention, which someone else was obviously getting now. When he did finally come into my room, he apologized for the long wait. He explained that he just saw a young lady, who was all by herself and had just been diagnosed with breast cancer. She was not turned away for lack of funds; Dr. Beird was going to find a way to make things happen. He spent a lot of time reassuring her.

I told him that I understood, and that he has always given me all the time I needed and treated me like a person and not a number. He said "Well, you ARE a person."

I told him I knew that but some doctors have one foot in the door and one foot in the room. However, he always sat down to talk to me, and I appreciated that. I think that doctors need to hear that once in a while, when they feel like they are being pulled in many directions at the same time. I was so lucky to be dealing with all compassionate doctors who gave me as much time as I needed.

I had just seen Dr. Maresca, my breast surgeon. She spent nearly one hour with me just before my appointment with Dr. Beird, so I received extra time with her that day. We spent a lot of time discussing which drug I should be taking and weighing the pros and cons of each. We also discussed if I really needed to take follow-up drugs at all, since my tumor was so small, my lymph nodes were clean, and I chose the bilateral mastectomy. The test done on my tumor cells concluded that my chances of cancer recurring were 7%. According to Dr. Maresca, the *size* of my tumor was not taken into account in the test and therefore, I had a less than a 1% chance of the cancer returning.

Was it worth risking the side effects and paying thousands of dollars for medication when my risk factor was that low? I had so much to think about before making my final decision. I was still on the first three months of my new, expensive medication. I would be getting another three months worth of it through the mail soon. I had time to think about it, while finishing up the current medication.

I was already experiencing pains in my feet, which I thought was from going on the treadmill, but now I know it was a side effect from the anti-cancer drugs. I also had a bad back and knew that the anti-cancer drugs would cause osteoporosis. Did I want this? There was so much to think about.

My expansions were finished, and the time to wait from the last expansion to the "exchange surgery" was three weeks away, yet I was still getting letters of encouragement. Each time I would send out "updates," friends and family would respond. One of my Red Hat friends, Kaye, wrote the following:

> *Elaine,*
>
> *So glad to hear the good news. It's amazing the path our lives take. Who would have ever guessed you were at this crossroad? Perhaps it's a good thing we can't see the future, and thank God for our parents, who gave us a religion that we could turn to when times get tough.—K*

When I asked her if I could quote her in my book she said:

> *Elaine,*
>
> *Of course you can use my name and quote. Just glad to say something—anything to help you through this. We stand by so helplessly and wish there were more we could do. I'm so glad you are writing a book. There is bound to be many more women that will travel your path and will be looking for every little bit of encouragement they can get. Who better to offer it than someone who has already been there?—K*

I also felt the urgency to share what I had learned along my journey with others; who were going through the same thing, or knew someone who was going through what I was going through. I especially wanted to reach those who had no medical background. We all need someone or somewhere to go for information and support in times like these.

On March 3rd, I went to my plastic surgeon's office to meet with Dee Ann. We discussed the surgery; she answered my list of questions; and then we filled out the necessary paper. I also signed the sheet, giving permission to use the silicone implants and to be in a ten-year study, which was to ensure the safety of the implants.

Dee Ann was so easy to talk to. I cried a little as I reminisced with her about the day of my mastectomy and how Dr. Maresca stood by my side in the pre-op room, holding my hand, as the nurse was starting my IV. Dee Ann looked at me with such understanding eyes. She gave me a tissue, and I wiped my tears. I thank God for directing me to Dr. Maresca, Dr. Beird, and Dee Ann. They made such a difference in my journey.

Dee Ann gave me a "good luck" hug before I left. My hard expanders were felt by both of us, as we hugged. I told her that the next time I saw her, I would give her a "soft hug" because I was getting rid of the rocks that I had been carrying around. She smiled and agreed. Soon I wouldn't have to be embarrassed to hug again. I was so ready to have that final surgery.

The day before my surgery, e-mails and phone calls kept coming in. I felt so covered with prayer. One of the e-mails I received was from my nephew Brad (one of Marge's sons) who was helping to edit my book. He shared the beautiful story of when his infant son, Joshua, was about to go through surgery to remove one of his kidneys due to a cancerous tumor. He was in Joshua's hospital room praying over him while he lay in that metal crib that looked more like a prison cell. In the darkness of the room, barely lit by a small night light, Brad cried out to God in earnest prayer.

It was then that Brad heard God more clearly than he ever had before, as he heard God say, "Ask whatever you want and I will give it to you."

At that moment, Brad received a gift of faith to believe that God would bring his son through the surgery and all the events that would follow. Brad was able to share his faith with his family and friends by declaring that victory even before he saw it. He shared, "When you receive this gift for a particular time, there is no striving on your part. You don't beg or hope that God will answer your prayer—somehow, you just know he will."

I wrote back to Brad and thanked him for sharing that story. I told him that I was so at peace his time. I had no fear whatsoever. I told him that I was totally trusting in God. I also told Brad that I knew that there is always a risk in any surgery, but I was not afraid. I had grown so much through what I had gone through so far. It was so different this time.

I also told him that if for some reason, something goes wrong, I just want to make sure that my book gets finished to help educate other women out there, who have to face breast cancer and feel unprepared. I told him that I just have to add the last surgery and my story would be complete.

I knew that I could trust that Brad would honor my request. He knew that I grew in my faith throughout my illness, as he did during Joshua's illness and recovery. We both want to share our stories to help others, who may be like I was the first time around. I was trying to control everything around me. The sooner we all let go and trust that God is there to take care of us, the easier it is for us to endure whatever we have to.

I thanked Brad for helping me with my book. He and I formed a special bond by working together to tell my story. Everything happens for a reason.

Brad wrote back and said,

Aunt Elaine,

God is good! The reason why things all work out in the long run is because they are orchestrated by Jesus to give God the glory. God allowed you to go through this trial and encounter those "bumps in the road" and is giving you a chance to write about it. He is doing all this for a reason. Romans 8:28 says, "And we know that all things work together for good to those who love God, to those who are called according to His purpose" (NKJV).

Aunt Elaine, you know that you love God, and I hope you know that you are called by God through this season in your life. He is giving you an amazing opportunity to share your faith-filled words and experiences with others so they can be blessed and God will be glorified. ALL THINGS work together for good! ALL THINGS!

Be blessed,

Love,
Brad and Family

CHAPTER 8

The Final Surgery— "The Exchange"

❋

I WENT TO SURGERY THE next day and was so calm and ready to have my last surgery. My blood pressure was 120/68. The anesthesiologist asked me if I was nervous. I said, "No! I am SO ready to get this over with." He looked at me and smiled and knew that I would be okay.

The expanders were removed and the silicone implants were put in. Everything went well except for the nausea and vomiting after surgery. However, after one day, I was feeling good again and was up and about. Now, all I had to do was to recover from that surgery and continue healing. The worst was in the past.

I still would have time to decide on whether or not I want to go through the nipple reconstruction. If I did, I would have to wait at least a couple of months for the incisions to heal. The tattoo part of the nipple would go over part of the scar from the incision. Also, the implants needed to fall more, before the nipple reconstruction.

When I talked to Dee Ann two days before my last surgery, she told me that some women don't have the nipple reconstruction and some do. Some women feel something is missing when they look into the mirror, so when they have the nipples done, it gives them a type of closure and allows them to go on with their lives. The choice would be totally up to me.

After my final surgery, I experienced some unexpected feelings. I could feel my silicone implants pressing against my chest wall. It felt like they were being held there with suction cups. My chest muscles were going into spasms again. The muscles, being tight, caused the front of my breasts to appear flat. I also felt the silicone implants going into my armpits. *Was this normal for this part of the recovery?* I did not want to feel my breasts 24/7. This was not what I expected to occur after the final surgery.

I asked my nurse neighbor what she thought about it. She suggested that I talk to someone who has been through it already so I e-mailed Heather and this was her answer:

> *Yes, this is normal. I think part of it is the awareness of them being different. Kind of like wearing a ring on a finger you don't normally wear it on. You will probably still feel the implants in your armpits for a month or two. One day you will just realize that they are no longer bothering you. Of course, if you just blocked it out on your mind there would be no problem…Easier said than done, but yes, everything is normal and your skin needs to continue to stretch. I do not feel mine at all anymore or notice that they are different from what my real breasts were like. The "suction cup feeling" will go away as things start to heal in there and some scar tissue forms to help hold them in.*
>
> *Heather*

I was so relieved to get this encouragement and agreed that I was only six days out of the surgery. I still had a lot of swelling and had to allow time for a complete healing.

It's important to remember that getting used to these new breasts will also take time. They will never be the same as before but are still covered with your skin, which has the ability to feel sensations and caresses. Once they are healed and the pain is gone, there is no reason to fear intimacy again.

Some women are so busy going from surgery to surgery that they actually go through a depression after the final surgery, when they realize that this is "as good as it is going to get." In some ways it may be necessary to say "Good-bye," to your old breasts and accept the new ones as "normal" from now on. That might require a period of mourning, but that's okay. Once you have allowed yourself to mourn that loss, you will be in a better frame of mind to accept what you have and go on.

I constantly remind myself that I have my life and my family which are more important than my breasts. I'd rather mourn the loss of my breasts than the loss of my loved ones. Many women, who have lost a family member, would gladly trade places with me. There IS life after a mastectomy. My faith helped me to put things in perspective, but I can't say that I did it without tears once in a while.

I have traveled the long journey and came through it a changed person. I feel that I have grown in faith and in character. I am stronger than I thought I was. All of these changes came as a result of going through a crisis in my life. The love and prayers of so many people helped me along the path of my journey and contributed to my recovery.

As I traveled on the path of my journey, I was convinced that it is in these difficult times that we grow spiritually. When things are going along well, it's easy to become complacent and feel that life is good and will continue to be good. However, it just takes an experience like having cancer that can either draw you closer to God or cause you to pull away. I decided to use this as a growing experience and was rewarded a hundred times over.

Until I was diagnosed with breast cancer, we thought that we had a relatively clean health history, as far as breast cancer is concerned. My father's mother died of breast cancer at the age of 60, but breast cancer on my father's side is not as pertinent as breast cancer on my mother's side. My mother's sister developed breast cancer in her 80's, so she had a lumpectomy and radiation. She didn't even go through a mastectomy.

However, recently there were three more of us diagnosed with breast cancer. Our family health history changed drastically. What was happening? Fortunately, my identical twin sister just recently had a mammogram which showed nothing, but her doctor put her on a medication to block estrogen from bonding with cancer cells, in case there were any cancer cells starting to grow in her breasts. My twin sister had also been on hormone replacement therapy for nearly ten years, as I had. Was this the "monster?" Was it the estrogen in my hormone replacement therapy that was feeding the cancer in my body all the while?

We kept hearing that we're on the cutting edge of discovering the cause and cure for breast cancer. I hope that this is true. I was lucky in that I was diagnosed early in the disease process and I am cured. Everyone isn't as lucky as I am. I also believe that everything happens for a reason. I believe that God allowed me to go through this experience so that I could write about it and tell others how to navigate these waters. Everything happens for a reason, and I feel privileged to be able to accept that cross and go on to help others through my experience. I did not do it without spiritual help and the support of many people.

Remember the train that we are on during our lifetime and all the people that get on and off and stay for different periods of time? Well, God had to add many extra cars to my train, because so many people got on and stayed with me throughout my journey. I am so blessed.

As my train exited the tunnel, the light was shining brightly and a glorious God was there to rejoice with us. Do I wish that I had never gone through this difficult time in my life? I don't think so. Everything happens for a reason and we learn from all of those tough times. After the storm comes a rainbow. My rainbow is filled with beautiful colors and is breath-taking and life-giving. God is good!

CHAPTER 9

In a Nutshell

---※---

BEING A REGISTERED NURSE, I have always loved doing patient teaching. Keeping that in mind, I took advantage of an opportunity to do it in a concise way in this chapter.

Do Monthly Self-Breast Exams Religiously

If you feel a lump, go to your doctor as soon as possible. Don't procrastinate. It is not worth taking a chance, since it just MIGHT be cancer.

Start Your Annual Mammograms When Your Doctor Advises

Remember everyone doesn't need to start annual mammograms at the same age. Your family and your personal health history will dictate when you should start.

Follow up on any Abnormalities in Mammograms

If you feel that something isn't quite right, then that is reason enough to call for an appointment. Be vigilant about your appointments, exams and follow-up. Take your list of question with you to ALL appointments.

Any Change is a Good Enough Reason to Call Your Doctor

No one knows your breasts like you do. If something doesn't seem just right, call your doctor. Examine your breasts in different positions—lying down, sitting up, in the shower, in front of the mirror, etc. Remember that MOST cancerous lumps are hard, but not ALL. If you feel something different, get it checked out ASAP!

If You Are Diagnosed with Breast Cancer, Discuss Options

As the old saying goes, "There is more than one way to skin a cat." Discuss radiation, chemotherapy, and surgery. After gathering all your information, make an informed decision and don't look back. What is right for you may not be right for another woman with breast cancer.

Trust Your Doctor or Go for Another Opinion

If you don't trust or feel comfortable with your doctor, go for another opinion. It's difficult enough going through breast cancer. If you don't have confidence in your doctor, find another one. You are putting your life in your doctor's hands, so trusting your doctor is a MUST.

Keep a Journal for Proof that You are Making Progress

You will need these reminders when it seems like time is standing still. Comparing where you are to where you were can surprise you. Celebrate even the "baby steps."

Expect Bumps in the Road as You Go through Your Journey

If you are a type "A" personality, like I am, it takes time to accept the fact that everything will not go totally as planned or expected.

We all have setbacks but it's getting through those difficult times that makes us stronger and brings us closer to God.

Take One Day ay a Time

You can go crazy by looking at the whole picture. When you enter the tunnel of your journey, you cannot see the light at the end. However, if you take it one day at a time, you can find little (but achievable) goals to celebrate.

Keep Busy and Keep a Positive Attitude

Time will go by much faster if you keep your mind occupied and try to look at the glass as "half-full" instead of "half-empty." If you do this, when you reach the end of the tunnel, you will be able to rejoice and say, "I did it!" instead of "It's about time." Look around you and you will see many people who have it much worse than you do. Yet, even those people have good days.

It's All Right to Have a Good Cry

There are times when your cup overflows. Having a good cry can help get rid of the overflow and allow you to see your problems in a whole new perspective. We are all dealing with a "full plate" at times. When someone or something adds one more thing, it can bring on the tears. That's all right. We all need to "let it out" one way or another.

Be Aware of How Your Illness is Affecting Young Children

Your children and/or grandchildren are all affected by your illness. Most of them know that cancer is a bad disease. They may be afraid to hug you for fear of hurting you. Let them know how much their hugs help you feel better. They need to know that they make a difference in your recovery.

Plan on Doing Things while You are on Your Journey

On days that you are feeling good, make time for fun. You don't have to go on a trip, like we did, but going out for dinner or taking a ride in the car will at least get you out of the house. It's amazing how much better you feel after a little outgoing.

Expect to Have Muscle Spasms During the Reconstruction

Remember, your muscles are suffering also, as they are being stretched. They will rebel at first by going into a spasm, but that will settle down in time. You may find that using an over-the-counter painkiller will help you tolerate these spasms. If that does not help, ask your doctor for a muscle relaxant.

Do NOT Use a Heating Pad for Muscle Spasms

Your skin is being stretched as well as the muscles. This skin is very thin and delicate. The nerve receptors for hot and cold are no longer there, so you can get a third-degree burn without feeling anything happening.

It Takes Time to Accept Your New Breasts

Your new breasts are never going to be like your original breasts, but they are yours and are covered with skin so you can still feel being touched. After the healing is complete and the pain is gone, it's all right to be intimate again. It may take time to mourn the loss of your old breasts before you can accept the new ones, but that's okay.

The Exchange surgery is Not the End of Your Journey

After the exchange, there is still a lot of healing to take place before your new breasts feel normal to you. The "suction cup" feeling on your chest wall and the spongy feeling in your armpits will go away as healing and stretching of the skin and the muscle is complete.

Let Go and Let God

The sooner you learn to let go of control and let God help you through your trying days, the better off you will be. "Letting go and letting God" is NOT a sign of weakness, but rather a sign of FAITH. I decided to use this as a time to grow in my faith and I was rewarded a hundred times over.

Remember the old sayings, "It's in the valleys that we grow" or "No pain, no gain." I certainly found this to be so true. During my journey of dealing with cancer, a double mastectomy, reconstruction, and all the pain and suffering that goes with it, I have grown in character and in my faith. During this time, I received several e-mails from Sadonna, a friend of mine, who regularly sends out prayer requests and updates. In one of her e-mails, she included a poem, which I read over many times because it had so much meaning to me. It talked about how pain is a necessary part of life, because in seasons of discomfort, we seek God more often. If we didn't have pain or distress, would we still seek Him? Certainly, pain is never enjoyable, but it did lead me to call out to God, and He answered me with a resounding chorus of peace, love, and support.

CHAPTER 10

A Husband's Perspective

By Ron Embrey

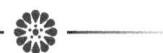

As I was getting towards the end of my book, I was taking a shower one morning, where I do a lot of my deep thinking, and I almost heard a voice talking to me. It seemed to be saying, "We need to hear from the other one who traveled this journey with you—we need to hear Ron's story."

I could hardly wait to get out of the shower to tell Ron that it was important to hear his voice, too. I told him that my story would be much more complete if he would be willing to tell the story from a husband's perspective. I knew that he went through his own agonies and his voice needed to be heard, as well as mine. Ron said, "I could do that."

I cried as I told Ron that this story isn't just about me. It's also about what he had to endure and accept along the way. I wanted him to tell what he experienced along OUR journey. I acknowledged the fact that he had his own struggles, while he was trying to help me through mine. He would benefit by getting his feelings out on paper also and then we would be able to go off together to our "living happily ever after" ending. This is what he wrote:

The last year has been a real roller coaster ride. We sold our condo at Greenview Place in March, 2008 by cell phone and fax machine on our way to Florida. While in Florida, we signed a purchase Agreement for our new condo at Shadows On The Green. On May 6th, we moved out of our Greenview condo and stored our furniture for two days on the moving van. Finally, on May 8th, we moved into our dream condo and enjoyed setting up housekeeping in our "new digs." Life was good for a while, but then the wheels started to come off the wagon.

Elaine had her annual mammogram on Jun 2nd, a pretty routine but painful procedure for her. The radiologist saw something that she felt needed follow-up. This suspicious area had been seen before and was being watched, but this time, watching wasn't good enough. A biopsy was suggested.

Elaine's gynecologist made an appointment for her with Dr. Carlotta Maresca, a breast surgeon. On July 2nd, we both went to Dr. Maresca's office for the pre-op visit. I was with Elaine when the doctor said she felt a lump and it needed to come out ASAP. I felt the blood drain from my body.

What in the world was going on? We were used to being in control. Our plans and dreams were being dashed on the rocks. We tried to keep our composure, but inside, we were in turmoil. Was I in the beginning stages of losing my wife? What would I do by myself? Elaine was (and is) the focal point of my life. Maybe she will be able to put this all in prespective. I sure hope so. We have profound respect for our physicians and their ability to fix us when we're broken. With God's help, all would eventually be okay. Wouldn't it?

A lumpectomy was scheduled for July 31st. Marge, Elaine's sister, and her Aunt Helen were at the surgery center with us when Dr. Maresca came to the recovery room after the surgery. The look on her face told us that the news wasn't good. She said the lump contained abnormal cells. When questioned further, she agreed that she expected it to be malignant.

This was NOT what we expected. We were confident that we would leave the surgery center happy that day, knowing that we just had a scare but that all would be okay, as Elaine kept telling everyone. WRONG! I was not prepared for this shock. My mind was spinning as I wondered what was in store for us.

After a follow-up visit with Dr. Maresca on August 18th, Elaine was scheduled for a double mastectomy two days later. Things were moving fast, WAY TOO FAST! We were going through the motions of a normal life, but we knew we were heading into uncharted waters for us.

Nurse Elaine had always taken care of our family's health and we were lucky. She always made decisions based on her experience and training that carried us through emergencies. Now our *nurse* was the *patient*. How would I cope with her pain and suffering? I knew I couldn't do it alone. We had a large group of friends and relatives praying for Elaine and me. We felt their support but would it be enough? Being retired, I had all the time in the world to try to take care of Elaine. I hoped I had the strength and wisdom to do and say the right things.

We discussed our situation the night before our visit with Dr. Maresca. Elaine decided that she wanted both breasts removed, even though she knew the cancer was only in one. She also did not feel it was necessary to have breast reconstruction. I agreed with all her decisions, as I truly wanted her to be happy with the outcome. However, Dr. Maresca changed her mind.

Dr. Maresca told Elaine that she was still young and she feared that Elaine would not be happy with her looks if she merely had her breasts removed. She told Elaine that she knew she cared about how she looked and reconstruction would allow her to feel "more normal" afterwards.

She then looked at me and asked how I felt about it. I told her that we had actually discussed it the night before, and I told Elaine that I would agree with whatever decision she made. I just wanted her to be happy with her decision and with the outcome. I could not tell her what she should do. I was Elaine's husband but it was HER body. She had to be sure that she would be satisfied with reconstruction, ready to deal with the extensive time this would take and ultimately, decide if it was all worth it. I wanted her to know that I would support her with any decision she made. Since Dr. Maresca had been through breast cancer and reconstruction herself, we talked about it for a while and then Elaine decided to take her advice and have the reconstruction.

Somehow we made it to the surgery day. We hugged and cried together before leaving for the hospital. We knew that she would never be the same, but we had to get rid of the cancer. I was scared for Elaine. She was being strong, but I knew she wanted to scream out, "Why me, God?" I was trying to be strong for her. However, when our parish priest, Fr. Bert, visited us the day of surgery to anoint Elaine, I lost it. She was the one needing surgery, but I ended up sobbing and begging for help.

Many had gone through this before Elaine and survived. However, this was my wife. I never thought we would have to deal with cancer. We were always faithful with our doctor appointments and check-ups. I guess that is why this cancer was caught in the early stages. Dr. Maresca said it could have been there for ten years before the lump was large enough to feel. Elaine did not deserve this but we both knew that we had been blessed with good health for almost 65 years and that maybe the message here was that this could be construed to be a positive event. Many others have not been so lucky and paid the ultimate price long before their time. We would beat the beast!

Dr. Maresca removed both breasts and Dr. Beird inserted the tissue expanders as part of the reconstruction process. After surgery, Marge and I waited for what seemed like an eternity for news from the recovery room. We eventually found out that Elaine had been in the recovery room for several hours and they were just waiting for a room. Nobody told us that. We finally had to press for more information and ask to see her. We did not need this additional stress.

As I approached the information desk for the second time, I'm afraid the look on my face exposed my true feelings at that point. I was tired, frustrated and angry about the way we, as relatives of the patient, were being treated. Doesn't anyone care about us? With all the staff sitting around, there must be someone who has time to periodically give us an update. Dozens of others in the waiting room were going through the same anxious moments, concerned about their loved ones.

Our son from Troy, a suburb of Detroit, was due to arrive at the hospital around 7:00 p.m. to see his mother. We joked, "Just wait until 'Detroit' gets here! Heads will roll." They said that she would be in her room soon. After over seven hours, we finally were told we could go to her room to see her.

As we entered the room we could see that Elaine was very groggy. At least the worst was over, or so I thought. As the evening wore on, Elaine made little progress trying to get the drugs out of her system. I wished I could have taken her place many times to relieve her of her pain and discomfort.

The next day Elaine was discharged. I felt so helpless as I went to get the car to bring her home. A taxi driver could have done that. It didn't do any good to dwell on my frustrations. I had a job to do, however small, and after all, I was not the issue here. Elaine needed me and I needed to be there for her. I brought her home on the day after surgery. She really needed another day to recover but we weren't given that option. Eventually, Marge and I decided we could do better for Elaine if she were home.

I had to learn how to change Elaine's dressings and remove the collected fluids from the drains. I never thought I could deal with this, but somehow I did. My wife needed me and I did my best to take care of her. That was the least I could do. After all, she had been taking care of me for over forty years.

The expanders were scheduled to come out and the permanent implants put in on March 5th. The waiting was finally over. No more saline injections to inflate the expanders. No more pain and discomfort from those temporary balloons.

The implants are finally in and Elaine's body is adjusting. It's still new territory and we don't know much about the final outcome other than what others tell us. We are learning little by little and day by day.

All I know is that my wife had cancer and beat it. She has been a real trooper through this whole process. I doubt I would handle it as well. We believe we have many years ahead of us to live and enjoy to the fullest. We are looking at life with a whole new outlook that involves family and friends and our church. We have been blessed with new life. I thank God for returning my wife to me, and I know we will enjoy many fun-filled years looking out at the deer and golfers from our dream condo on the golf course.

EPILOGUE

Everything is More Precious Now

After my final surgery (the exchange), I sent out an "Update on Elaine" to several friends and relatives. This time I included the grandchildren, who have e-mail addresses. They were all praying for me and hoping that I would get better soon.

Morgan (10 1/2 years old) and I have been e-mailing back and forth for the last several months. Since we don't get to see our Grand Rapids grandchildren as often as we'd like, the computer age had helped Morgan and me to form a bond by sharing what's in our minds and in our hearts via e-mails. That is very special to me. Ron also mentioned several times that he is so glad that we have this relationship.

Kassidy, (10 years old) occasionally sends an e-mail also but she is very busy with her traveling soccer team. I know that she is thinking and praying for me often. When I do get to see her, she comes to give me those love-filled hugs that grandmas need. She somehow found time to make all of us homemade scarves for

Christmas. She knows that I'm a Red Hatter, so she made mine in purple and red. I wore it to a recent soccer game of hers. She smiled when she saw it. That made my day.

Aaron (7 years old) is usually quiet around us, but I know that he is concerned about me and that he loves me. When we were at their Grand Rapids home recently, I asked him and his sister Morgan if I could mention them in my book and share what they wrote to me (in their get well cards) after my first surgery. Their eyes lit up and they both gave their permission. I wanted them to know that their love and support helped me to get better.

Brandan (11 1/2 years old) is our oldest grandchild and is the "deep thinker." I just know that my illness had a much bigger effect on him than I originally realized. He usually calls his grandpa to talk to him about whatever sporting event he is attending at the time. However, after my final surgery and in response to my "Update on Elaine" e-mail to him, he called ME one evening. When I answered the phone, I heard this quiet, very concerned voice, saying, "Hi Grandma. How are you doing?" I could tell he was worried.

I told Brendan that I was doing fine and I was feeling a little better each day. He knew that healing would take time, but he just needed to hear his grandma's voice. He asked me about my book and what kind of software I was using to write it. We talked about my book, what he was doing at his school and about his sports. We were on the phone for almost an hour just chatting. Then he said, "Grandma, I have to go now." I thanked him for calling and told him that I loved him. He said, "I love you too." That boy will never know how much his phone call meant to me. He didn't ask to talk to Grandpa this time. He needed his grandma that day and I needed him.

Brady (age 5 1/2) is always happy to see us. He doesn't realize what I actually went through, so when he hits the front door, he comes charging toward us and jumps into our arms to give us big hugs. Todd (his dad) frequently reminds him that Grandma just had surgery. He tells him to be gentle. We give the little ones just enough information for their ages. When they see me, they see their "Grandma" and that is all they see, so they act like they have always acted…they run to us for those hugs.

Brooke Elaina, my namesake, (age 4) has no idea what I went through. I'm glad that she doesn't understand because I'm just her "same old Grandma" that I was before. She climbs up on my lap and brings a handful of books with her and wants me to read. I read to her until she falls asleep in my arms and then I carry her to her bed and tuck her in. Each time I do this I experience "a little bit of heaven." I just cannot get enough of those loving grandchildren.

As a result of the cancer, surgeries, pain and adjustments I experienced recently, I now have a whole new lease on life. Everything is more precious to me. My journey down this new path has transformed me. It's very hard to explain but I now realize the meaning of the saying " Every cloud has a silver lining."

Shortly after my double mastectomy, and after we found out that my lymph nodes were clean (meaning that they removed all the cancer and I was cured), I was a changed person. A few days after my surgery, I got up before daylight, went out on our deck overlooking the golf course, and took pictures of the sun rising. It was actually a spiritual moment in my life. The sun glowed like a ball of fire; the birds' singing never sounded so beautiful; and the frogs even seemed to be rejoicing with me on that God-filled morning. When our contractor asked me later that day if life is any different now, I said, "Yes, I was up taking pictures of the sun rising this morning." He smiled.

During the time of my battle with cancer and then my recovery, my twin sister managed to sell her house in town and moved into the brand new condo right next door to us. She had lost her husband three years earlier and was ready to give up the big house, the pool, and the huge yard. Miraculously, the condo right next to us was the only one available to buy in our new condo complex at that time. There would now be three of us to look out for each other as our health and family needs dictated. I know that it is just one more blessing that God has bestowed on all of us. As the saying goes, "When God closes a door, He opens a window." When we were little, my twin and I used to talk about growing up, getting married, and living in a duplex together. Our childhood dream has come true.

Glossary

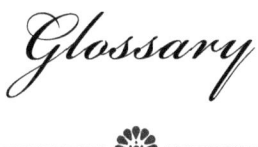

benign: not cancer; not malignant

biopsy: removing a sample tissue to see whether cancer cells are present

bilateral: on both sides of the body

breast implant: a sac used to increase breast size or restore the shape of the breast after a mastectomy. The sac is filled with silicone gel (a synthetic material) or sterile saltwater (saline)

cancer: It is not just one disease but rather a group of diseases. All forms of cancer cause cells in the body to change and grow our of control. Most types of cancer cells form a lump or mass called a tumor, which can invade and destroy healthy tissue.

carcinoma: a malignant tumor that begins in the lining layer (epithelial cells) of organs. At least 80% of all cancers are carcinomas, and almost all breast cancers are carcinomas.

carcinoma in situ: an early stage of cancer, in which the tumor is still only in the structures of the organ where it first started. The disease has not invaded other parts of the organ or spread to distant parts of the body. Most in situ carcinomas are highly curable.

chemotherapy: treatment with drugs to destroy cancer cells; most of the time called just "chemo." Chemotherapy is often used in addition to surgery or radiation to treat cancer when it has spread, when it has come back (recurred, or when there is a strong chance that it could recur.

cyst: a fluid-filled mass that is usually not cancerous. A needle aspiration can be done to remove the fluid for testing.

dense: thick, compact

diagnosis: identification of a disease by its signs or symptoms and through the use of imaging tests and lab findings

estrogen: a female sex hormone produced mainly by the ovaries and in smaller amounts by the adrenal glands. In women, levels of estrogen and other hormones work together to regulate the development of secondary sex characteristics, including the breasts. In breast cancer, estrogen may promote the growth of cancer cells.

estrogen receptors: molecules that function as a cell's "welcome mat" for estrogen circulating in the blood. Cancers with estrogen receptors (ER-positive) are more likely to respond to hormonal therapy.

expansion: an enlargement, increase, etc.

fibrocystic changes (fibrocystic disease): a term that describes certain benign changes in the breast. Symptoms of this condition are breast swelling or pain. The breasts often feel lumpy or nodular.

hormone replacement therapy (HRT): the use of estrogen and progesterone from an outside source after the body has stopped making its own supply because of natural or induced menopause.

hyperplasia: an abnormal increase in the number of cells in a specific area, such as the lining of the breast ducts or the lobules. By itself, hyperplasia is not cancerous, but when the increase is obvious and/or the cells are atypical (unlike normal cells), the risk of cancer developing is greater."

incisions: a cut made with a knife, expecially for surgical purposes

inflammatory breast disease (inflammatory carcinoma): a type of invasive breast cancer that spreads to lymphatic vessels in the skin covering the breast. The skin of the affected breast is red, feels warm, and may thicken to the consistency of an orange peel.

invasive ductal carcinoma; a cancer that starts in the milk passages (ducts) of the breast and then breaks through the duct wall, where it invades the fatty issue of the breast. When it reaches this point, it has the potential to spread (metastasize) elsewhere in the breast, as well as to other parts of the body through the bloodstream and lymphatic system. Invasive ductal carcinoma is the most common type of breast cancer, accounting for about 80% of breast malignancies. (Also known as infiltrating ductal carcinoma)

jaundice: a condition characterized by yellowness of skin, whiteness of eyes, mucuos membranes, and body fluids, due to deposition of bile pigment resulting from excess bilirubin in the blood.

lipoma: a fatty tumor. They are frequently multiple, but not metastatic.

lump: any kind of mass in the breast or elsewhere in the body that may be cancerous or not

lumpectomy: surgery to remove the breast tumor and a small amount of surrounding normal tissue

lymph nodes: small, bean-shaped collections of immune system tissue, such as lymphocytes, found along lymphatic vessels. They remove cell waste, germs and other harmful substances from lymph. They help fight infections and also have a role in fighting cancer.

malignant: cancerous

mammogram: an x-ray of the breast; a method of detecting breast cancers that cannot be felt: Mammograms are done with a special type of x-ray machine that is used only for this purpose. A mammogram can show a developing breast tumor before it is large enough to be felt by a woman or even by a highly skilled health care professional.

mastectomy: surgery to remove all or part of the breast, and sometimes other tissue

metastasize: to spread from one part of the body to another

magnetic resonance imagine (MRI): a method of taking pictures of the inside of the body; Instead of using x-rays, MRI uses a powerful magnet to send radio waves through the body; the images appear on a computer screen as well as on film.

needle localization: a procedure used to guide a surgical breast biopsy when the lump is hard to locate or when there are areas that look suspicious on the mammogram but there is not a distinct lump. In this procedure, a thin needle is placed into the breast. X-rays are then used to guide the needle to the suspicious area. The surgeon then uses the path of the needle as a guide to locate the abnormal area to be removed.

oncologist: a doctor with special training in the diagnosis and treatment of cancer

Pap Smear (Pap Test): A test to detect cancer in smears of bodily secretions, especially from the cervix and the vagina.

pathologist: a doctor who specializes in the diagnosis and classification of diseases by lab tests, such as examining tissue and cells under a microscope. The pathologist determines whether a tumor is benign or cancerous and, if cancerous, the exact cell type and grade.

prognosis: a prediction of the course of a disease; the outlook for the chances of survival. For example, women with breast cancer that was detected early and who received prompt treatment have a good prognosis.

prosthesis: an artificial part used to replace or improve the function of a body part. For example, a breast prosthesis can be worn under the clothing after a mastectomy.

radiation: high energy particles that are used for x-rays and in higher doses in cancer treatment. Natural radiation comes from radon gas and from sources in outer space, such as the sun.

radiology technician (radiation therapist): a person with special training to operate the equipment that delivers radiation therapy

reconstructive mammoplasty (breast recostruction): plastic surgery that is done after mastectomy to rebuild the breast

re-excision: a second surgery to remove remaining cancer. This may be done if cancer cells were found at the edge of surgically removed tissue.

silicone gel: synthetic material used in breast implants. Because of its flexibility, strength and texture, it is similar to the natural breast.

surgery: the treatment of disease, injury, etc. by manual or instrumental operations.

tumor: an abnormal lump or mass of tissue. Tumors can be benign (not cancerous) or malignant (cancerous).

ultrasound (sonography, ultrasonography): an imaging method in which high-frequency sound waves are used to outline a part of the body. The sound wave echoes are picked up and displayed on a monitor (similar to a television screen). This painless method is sometimes useful in distinguishing fluid-filled cysts from solid tumors. It can also be used to guide a needle biopsy of breast abnormalities too small to feel.

RECOMMENDED RESOURCES

Cancer Information Websites

American Cancer Society

    www.cancer.org

    (800) 227-2345

This site provides information on cancer, support resources, and research. Upon request, the American Cancer Society will provide you with a free kit to help you learn about cancer and organize your health care information. This kit will help you to keep track of test results, doctor appointments, and medicines, and assist you in talking with doctors and nursed

Cancer Care Incorporated

    www.cancercareinc.org

    (800) 913-4673

This site provides chat rooms.

Leukemia Society of America

www.leukemia.org
(800) 955-4572

This site provides information about leukemia, lymphoma, Hodgkin's disease, and myeloma.

National Breast Cancer Coalition

www.natlbcc.org
(202) 296-7477

This site provides information about the fight against breast cancer.

National Cancer Institute

www.nci.nih.gov
(800) 422-6237

This site includes information about clinical trials, and education about many different types of cancer.

National Coalition for Cancer Survivorship

www.cansearch.org
(877) 622-7937

Advocacy organization for cancer survivors

National Lymphedema Network

www.lymphnet.org
(800) 541-3259

This site provides education on lymphedema.

OncoLink

>www.oncolink.upenn.edu

This site provides updates on treatments and advances.

Oncotype DX

>www.oncotypeDX.com

This site includes information on a test to determine your chances of cancer recurring.

Patient Resource publishing

>www.patientresource.net

This site contains an exhaustive collection of resources including: cancer education, cancer support and advocacy groups, credible cancer resources, inspirational survivor stories, clinical trials, and many more related websites.

Susan G. Komen Foundation

>www.breastcancerinfo.com
>(800) 462-9273

This site contains news and stories about cancer survivors.

Recommended Reading

Breast Cancer: What You Need to Know Before Treatment. Publication DCH-1234. (2003). Michigan Department of Community
Health: Cancer Prevention and Control Section, Lansing, MI Additional copies can be ordered from Michigan Department of Community Health

Bureau of Health Policy Regulations and Professions
Attn: Carmen Wiggins
P.O. Box 30454
Lansing, MI 48909
Phone: (517) 335-1763
Fax: 517-335-4886

Brown, Zora & Boatman, Karl. (2009). 100 Questions & Answers About Breast Cancer. 3rd Edition. Jones and Bartlett Publishing, LLC. Sudbury, MA.

Cancer Resource Guide: 2008 Edition. (2008). Cure: Cancer Updates, Research & Education. Dallas, TX. www.curetoday.com

Patient Resource Cancer Guide: A treatment and facilities guide for patients and their families. (2008). Fall/Winter 2008 Edition. Patient Resource Publishing. Parkville: MO. www.patientresourses.net

Sorenson, Sharon &Metzger, Suzanne. (2000). The Complete Idiot's Guide to Living with Breast Cancer. Alpha Books. MacMillan USA, inc. Indianapolis, IN.

Steligo, Kathy. (2005). The Breast Reconstruction Guidebook: Issues and answers from research to recovery. Carlo Press. San Carlos, CA.

Your Surgery Planner: Reconstruction surgery with silicone gel-filled breast implants. (2006). Allergan, Inc. Santa Barbara, CA 93111. www.allergan.com

Bibliography

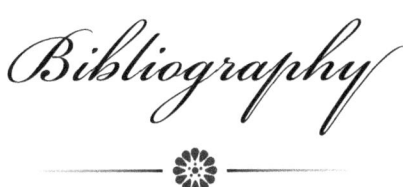

Breast Cancer Dictionary. (2006). American Cancer Society, Inc. No. 467500—Revised 10/07

New American Webster Handy College Dictionary, The. New Third Edition. (Eds.) Albert and Loy Morehead. (1995. Penguin Books. New York, NY.

Taber, Clarence. Taber's Cyclopedic Medical Dictionary. Eighth Edition. (1961). F.A. Davis Company. Philadelphia, PA.

ELAINE EMBREY, R.N.

Breast Cancer

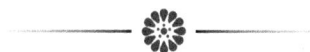

"ON THE MORNING OF surgery, Ron came into the bathroom as I was getting dressed, took one look at me and knew that this was a difficult time for me, seeing my red eyes from crying so hard. Without saying a word, he took me into his arms and held me close, as we both burst into tears. I felt his body shaking as I'm sure he felt mine. We just stood there sobbing and holding each other. We both needed that. We had been strong for each other long enough. Now, it was time to let it all out. It was so cleansing. I thank God for that moment and for a man who loves me enough to cry with me at a time like this."

Travel the path with a breast cancer patient and her husband as they take this courageous journey together. Elaine Embrey, R.N., gives an informative and detailed account from diagnosis through reconstruction and all the unexpected bumps in between. Elaine has the unique ability to take today's confusing medical terms and procedures and explain them clearly enough for anyone to understand. This book a "must have" for all who are looking for real answers on how to stand victorious through this challenge. Elaine's husband, Ron, also shares his perspective in a heart-tugging fashion which will help all friends and family members relate to a loved one in this situation.

Elaine Embrey is a retired Registered Nurse who survived breast cancer, and now lives with her husband, Ron, in Bay City, Michigan. While going though her journey, she grew in character and in her faith. She now feels compelled to share her story and everything she has learned along the way, in the hopes of helping others who have travel this same path.

As a result of the cancer, surgeries, pain and adjustments I experienced recently, I now have a new lease on life. Everything is more precious to me. My journey down this new path has transformed me. It's hard to explain but I now realize the meaning of the saying "Every cloud had a silver lining."

Shortly after my double mastectomy, and after we found out that my lymph nodes were clean (meaning that they removed all the cancer and I was cured), I was a changed person. A few days after that surgery, I got up before daylight, went out on our deck overlooking the golf course, and took pictures on the sun rising. It was actually a spiritual moment in my life. The sun glowed like a ball of fire; the birds' singing never sounded so beautiful; and the frogs even seemed to be rejoicing with me on that God-filled morning. When our contractor asked me later that day if life is any different now, I said, "Yes, I was up taking pictures of the sun rising this morning." He smiled.

During the time of my battle with cancer and then my recovery, my twin sister managed to sell her house in town and moved into the brand new condo right next door to us. She had lost her husband 3 years earlier and was ready to give up the big house, the pool, and the huge yard. Miraculously, the condo right next to us was the only one available to buy in our new condo complex at that time. There would now be three of us to look out for each other as our health and family needs dictated. I know that it is just one more blessing that God has bestowed on all of us, as the saying goes, "When God closes a door, He opens a window." When we were little, my twin and I used to talk about growing up, getting married, and living in a duplex together. Our childhood dream has come true.

www.ingramcontent.com/pod-product-compliance
Lightning Source LLC
LaVergne TN
LVHW012000070526
838202LV00054B/4977